I0464648

The Grim Reaper

Wears a White Coat

Michael D. Wylder

This book is dedicated to the physicians and other healthcare providers who see through the bullshit that is unfortunately the contemporary medical industrial complex. Any individual can 'buy into' and follow the path of the disease management system, go along, get along, and do nothing else.

I salute those with the courage to follow their heart, and keep the faith to treat others as they like to be treated. As long as individuals work primarily to acquire wealth and not improve their families, communities, and the world; the status quo shall prevail.

The story is 'fictional' the details are not. It is an invitation for those with the ability to help at the micro and macro societal levels to reconsider the current paradigm. Then create a better model focusing on health instead of disease management, on cooperation (building a better product for the greater good) instead of the competition (winner take all!).

With the current ACA, Affordable Healthcare Act, I recall paying two hundred fifty dollars for an antibiotic prescription that had cost twenty-three dollars before the mandatory healthcare coverage; same prescription at more than ten times the cost. The 'epi', epinephrine, pens made the news for their ten times rate increase, but practically all prescription costs increased! Also, with deductibles that range up to and beyond ten thousand dollars; how are individuals supposed to afford care? These are some of many examples, and proof that people's insatiable greed, not money, is the root of all evil. However, greed is a choice, and it can be changed as long as individuals remember it is up to them.

The lack of compassion in the contemporary medical model is ubiquitous. Profits for a relative few rather than better health for all is the guiding light.

Discussions of physician shortages require discernment. There are more students than ever. Medical schools are in the business to make money. Upon completion of my degree there were 19 Osteopathic medical schools, now there are 43. These schools create profits before physicians, and many do not find residency spots to complete their training.

Recently, I heard a news story that for the first time ever; the total number of students starting in Fall 2018 have over fifty percent of their students as women. In the contrived world we have, and live in day to day; this is neither an accident or coincidence.

The open, discerning mind has to ponder what legislation, trends, and healthcare policies are being prepared to roll out within the decade after they jump through the hoops of medical training.

Some of the students, regardless of their gender, are following a calling to service or are healers. Others are there for the prestige and salary. Far too many of the latter perpetuate the profession's shortcomings.

It is not a pleasant journey. Fear, greed, abuse, and a lack of compassion are the foundation of medical training. The current paradigm does not need another look; it needs to be rebuilt!

Allow me to step off the soapbox, and join Reginald as he continues his own journey.

Prologue

Reggie continues driving along the looping highway that surrounds and provides a circular access to all parts of the city; downtown, suburbia and all points in between and beyond. He does not feel like he should have any issues with breathing. However, he feels like he is smothering. He coughs, and forces some fast deep breathes. His air conditioner is working again, but he opts to lower the window, and drives with his arm resting upon the sun faded vinyl.

Feeling the salty perspiration roll down the medial side of his fibula; he follows the sensation as far as he can, until the salty wet stream is absorbed by his socks. He is in scrubs, and sneakers; his coat thrown hastily in the back seat earlier.

It's a relief to be able to feel something; even a small fleeting sensation, again. It's a pleasure to simply drive on the smooth highway, with the cruise control set one mile per hour over the speed limit in the sparse traffic. It's unlikely he will be bothered by law enforcement.

The thumping noise originating from the rear of his car has gone from constant

to an unpredictable, intermittent, before
shortly disappearing then resuming.
Checking his driver side view mirrors, he
doesn't think it's a tire issue. He
carefully changes lanes to see if it
returns; it does not appear to be a wheel
bearing or a tail pipe, but something is
noisy.

He looks up, his hands at the ten and
two o'clock positions on the steering
wheel, and glancing at his rear view mirror
with a stethoscope wrapped around behind it
dangling uneventfully. Looking into the
aging,frosted, reflective glass to see what
is behind him.

A commercial helps him realize the
radio is loud, and a practiced reach finds
the knob, and reduces the decibel level. A
glancing look at the vigilant digital clock
reminds him he has been driving around the
looping highway for an hour and a half.
What's confusing to him is he does not
realize the purpose nor the reason he is
driving around; so he continues; maybe
it'll come to him. He feels like he is in
the zone. He can wait.

Awakening

Journal Entry:

I am so tired. I wake up tired, all through the course of the day I'm tired, and I go to bed tired. I sometimes wonder how I make it through the days with attending physicians who are thinking you should be tired and stuporous as a ridiculous rite of passage...you do their H&Ps and scut work and they get to rest and have normal hours. It wouldn't be so bad, but they don't know how to communicate or teach effectively for that matter...they think their way is the best way, and they all tend to disparage others and their methods...I sometimes forget which attending I'm with.... Yet we are supposed to respect them, and tolerate their 'challenging' personalities and any character flaws they may have; after all they are the attending physicians...I am beyond glad that my time with Doctor Ashley is winding down...I fear I may go off on him...I'm running on adrenaline, my body feels like it is being slowly broke down and replaced with cyborg parts...I'm hungry all the time...the meals provided by the program do not provide much more than a quick break from the routine...they are processed, not fresh, or nutritious and do not quench the hunger pangs...I sometimes only feel numb and the walls of the hospital might as well be prison walls...at times it feels as if I'm a prisoner and marking time...awaiting the end of my sentence...I don't think I can describe to anyone what I have to go through; they don't understand...and my peers don't want to get past their own issues, let alone identify that someone else is also dealing with them...I'm in the midst of bustling activity; and I feel so alone... What have I got myself into?"

It's 5:15 AM and Reginald Myron Washington is not sure if he's awake or dreaming, or if the ringing he hears is from the bedside alarm clock. In this familiar dream he is facing a middle-aged man with a beige straw hat, denim overalls and scraggly beard framing a chubby face. The cherub face has green eyes glaring through rectangular, wire frame glasses. He's seen the character before in dreams as far back as he can remember; not every sleep event, but randomly present in his dreams.

"What the hell," is all he can manage to conjure through the sleepy foggy haze of his tired mind and body. "No way I've been asleep that long!" Groaning, he releases an exasperated sigh heard by no one else.

He notices he is in the same position he started nearly eight hours ago. He is tired both mentally and physically, and this is his new normal. However, normal does not mean desirable; especially in this case.

Thanks to a month long ER rotation, he reaches a whole new level of sleep deprivation. He doesn't like feeling tired all of the time; at times he feels like he is in a haze; other times a daze. Even the rare occurrence of eight hours of sleep does not recharge him. If he has a moment while commuting and sitting at a long line of traffic at a signal light; or in a chair he feels himself nodding off. This is in spite of copious amounts of caffeine.

His diet consists primarily of the

processed, institutional foods provided
by the hospital cafeteria. This is a
benefit included in the contract. This
nutrition depleted food is conveniently
available on site. This is the only
sustenance, unless it is interrupted by
an occasional real meal. Some of these
'real meals' are sponsored by the thirty
plus percent marketing budget of the
ambitious pharmaceutical companies. The
bottom line; the eating arrangement is
not sustaining him.

He takes a multi-vitamin; sometimes
twice a day, but is not confident he's
getting proper nutrition. He walks a lot
throughout the day, but a trip to the
gym to workout like he wants, and used
to be able is rare.

His life does not feel like it's
his own; he feels trapped. There is
nothing predictable, but the devious,
ominous, unpredictable and mind numbing
servitude. Staring at the white ceiling
looming silent, and textured over him; a
testimony to his commitment to persevere

and stay the tedious course he is on.

The view of the ceiling never changes, but it doesn't find fault with him either. As he fumbles for a switch on the bedside lamp with it's dusty shade another testimony to his personal commitment and priorities. He, as usual, has to wonder which day of the week it is. A deep breath is forced in order to give him motivation to start his day. "What the hell have I gotten myself into?" Posing that question to himself again; it's not the first time he truly ponders that question. Focusing his view, and looking at his phone's caller identification. It appears his mother, and a friend have called him. More times than not, he lacks the mental energy at the end of the day to return a call, let alone conduct a conversation.

He hopes they understand. The long days spent on his feet, and under the profession's heels, while in tow of an attending physician and other residents jockeying for position is deceptive.

You can lean against a wall or sit, but here is no time to relax your mind. There is always something to think about or the unknown question or situation you have to prepare to answer or encounter.

Also, being around people who are sick takes a toll on a healthy body. His hands are raw from the continuous hand-washing. He has been coughed upon, and smelled odors he did not think could emanate from a live human body. All of this with his sincere, and professional demeanor which provides an outer mask of tolerance and not a hint of his inner disgust. He doesn't feel like a robot, as they wouldn't feel tired or hungry. However, he does feel mechanical, as if he going through the motions at times.

Feeling isolated from family and friends is new. He cannot expect them to understand his day to day routine. He finds it difficult to explain the logic in the process of creating physicians when he does not understand it himself. He notices the profession lacks the element of empowering them to be autonomous and free thinkers. It cannot even promote health among its own ranks.

The profession successfully focuses on both luring and coercing them into the profession. It does this with the desires of technology, power, prestige and money on one hand. However, on the other hand, it effectively uses fear in it's most primitive forms to motivate and shape them. Like a frog in a pot of water that gets heated up ever so slowly; future physicians are created and molded in the turbulent waters of fear and mediocrity. The misinformed are leading the uninformed.

Reggie, as he likes to be called, is beyond feeling tired; he is being tired. As a resident physician, he has been sleep deprived for the past four years while at medical school. Between the two years of coursework and two, too busy clerkship years, good rest and nutrition have been eluding him. He often ponders the reasons a physician's

13

education is not salubrious and take into account how to keep the bodies that they mold and program in the training process more healthy. It certainly seems hypocritical that the hippocratic oath to do no harm is ignored. Sitting up, he dozes off again, but dropping a shoe awakens him. Being tired, and sleep deprived is indeed his his new normal.

Momentarily keeping his eyes closed, and quietly planning his day. The glow of the lamp sends a soft glow to his retinae. This morning he is expected to conduct patient rounds before the surgeon. He knows Doctor Ashley will arrive in a leisurely, but random time. He'll sense his presence as he sucks the calm off the units. As usual, he'll be abrasive in his demeanor and disrespectful to all the staff except for peer colleagues.

Reggie is disgusted with the mixed messages the attending physicians give him. It is a catch twenty-two that he and others find themselves as hapless participants in a game that they do not wish to play.

It's not correct to call the process a benign,rite of passage. In reality, it's systemic abuse, and indoctrination. The sometimes subtle misuse of power; and the overbearing process of overtly controlling others is dysfunctional, but accepted in many circles. Control the information; and alter rules on the fly creates an insecure mind; and ultimately controls the individual.

The game is insidious, and complex in its simplicity. It's a game of power and control. You can't make this stuff up! He is expected to examine the surgical site, interact with the patient, enter a note, but not actually manage the cases by adding or changing an order. He has many times been admonished, 'Don't change anything' when he attempts to manage the case.

Sound messed up? Well,it is. In the ethos of the schizophrenic world of medical education he receives a 'Why aren't you doing anything with the patient' when he follows the directive to not bother the case.

Heaven have mercy on you if you challenge them. The body of profession is bigger than the speck on a speck of dust, individual physician who wants to bravely challenge the status quo. This has been Reggie's world for the past five years. It takes a toll on the psyche and soul as he sometimes feels numb for hours at a time just to endure the commitment.

On routine cases, Doctor Ashley is a competent general surgeon. However, he is narcissistic and overbearing to the operating suite staff. In his opinion he always knows best. He has a string of failed marriages betray his lack of surgically precise interpersonal skills. He is in his element when he is in the surgical suite and in charge; to him the ideal world is an operating suite with his brand of oligarchy. Doctor Ashley also does not mind boldly tooting his own horn regarding his surgical skills. However, astute people realize he hand picks his cases and avoids anything out of the ordinary. In true denial, he fails to realize others despise him. In his own world thinking he's admired and respected.

Reginald tolerates him, and his personality, but despises his constant 'pimping'. Pimping sounds like a good idea at first glance. The benevolent attending physicians ask you questions that might be on a board exam; this can increase the resident's knowledge base and points to areas of review for further study. However, it can also be used as a forum to ask irrelevant, minutia not to increase the knowledge base, but to bully and intimidate. The motive is to remind the hapless young doctor who is the resident and who is the attending.

Reggie learns to especially despise the constant questions from Doctor

Asher. Discovering no matter what or how much you know, he continues until he asks Reggie a question that he can't answer. Nothing important, but minutia that's not likely easily found or researched or even useful. At times it can be a board exam question.

Ostensibly, he says its purpose is to increase knowledge, but more than likely it is present to establish the top dog standing in the hierarchy.

"Keep your eye on the prize," he thinks as he musters the mental and physical energy required to get out of bed and start this day. He is tired, and not energized by the prospect the day might bring. It wasn't always this way.

Reginald successfully completes an undergraduate degree in mechanical engineering from the flag ship state university. His costs covered by an academic scholarship. His primary mentor, Henry, guides him and provides wise counsel for his academic studies as well as funds. Advising him to fly joyfully under the radar, and to be discreet about his academic ambitions. Reggie started his college experience studying mechanical engineering. He met Henry after a sparsely attended lecture gave him the opportunity to ask him questions. Henry has an eye for talent and recognizes the potential in the polite,lanky lad asking the questions.

Henry, after listening to Reggie spouting off his youthful enthusiasm and innocence for two hours after the lecture over coffee and home made slices of apple pie al a mode with home made vanilla ice cream at a local diner; with sprinkled cinnamon and brown sugar providing a pleasant fragrance. It is a pleasant memory in his bank. It is there he got to know the humble scientist.

Henry is a scientist and intuitive soul, and he recognizes a healer's soul in Reginald's handshake and energy. He gets nothing but good vibes from his encounter and is just as delighted to spend time with young Reginald.

Henry surmises Reggie's interest in form and function and how dynamic systems interact that might bore him as an engineer. "You can easily parlay your interest in science and engineering into a career in medicine," he tells him.

Reggie listens intently and feels a warm, calm as his body and mind relaxes as he picks up on the sincerity of his message. "This guy is for real," he thinks. Reggie takes what he recommends to heart, and adds some biology and other prerequisite courses to his engineering degree. The way he figures it is he can have the degree he wants as well as the opportunity to become a physician. Either way he is following his passion; going in the flow.

He discusses his plans with Henry, and gets an affirmative nod. "I Like your plan," his handshake, and smile validate his words. "However, it's a cutthroat environment." Cautioning him, "If you are perceived as competition, there are students who will try to squash your spirit, and sabotage you."

When an optimistic positive individual such as Henry provides that wisdom, it carries a lot of weight. His sincerity shapes Reginald's view of the world that individuals may not always 'play fair'.

Reginald follows his passions and heeds Henry's guidance to follow his interests. He can still hear his voice say, "Follow your interests, that way you enjoy what you're doing all the time, and you end up where you need to be."

Reginald's parents are both math and science teachers at the local public high school. They encourage him to study and to pursue math and science courses. Inheriting their intellect, and their aptitude and soaking up their constant encouragement like a dry sponge takes in water.

Although they have the financial means; they chose not to spoil him with entitlement and selfishness. They choose to teach and demonstrate the qualities of selflessness and compassion; and not indulge his every want and desire. They do not put themselves in the position to give him 'things' to compensate for lack of emotional support.

They do this by example. They live modestly, and are not pretentious as they live beneath their means. They are courteous at home and in public and this is noticed by Reggie. They mind their own business, and do not seek conflict or drama; life has enough challenges without creating them.

The precocious Reggie notices these things at a young age. He's always been intuitive, empathic,and good at picking up the nonverbal cues from others around him. He has a knack of sensing others emotions and intentions; good or bad. He originally thought everyone was like him, but eventually learns that is not the case; many are too self-centered.

He also learns this discernment from them. He develops this as they discuss news events and simply do not accept things at face value. Reggie notices this is not how his friend's parents conduct themselves. He has always been attentive and able to read people and situations in an uncanny sixth sense sort of way.

He is a deep thinker and enjoys questioning things he observes everyday. His undergraduate degrees include mechanical engineering and philosophy. However, with an eye on the horizon; takes the required prerequisite courses of biology, chemistry, and physics as electives during summer school as Henry suggests.

During the summer school session, even the ambitious pre-med students are enjoying their off time, Reginald is not even a blip on their radar. A very focused, and dedicated student, he is not distracted by the festive atmosphere offered to the hormone driven, hedonistic, ambitious undergraduates.

He doesn't look down on them or

judge them for their behavior. It is just not his thing. He chooses to not use drugs or alcohol with the goal to numb himself. He realizes the training is numbing him out at times. He notices how often the very individuals who engage in such activities have less peace of mind than others. He surmises the biggest reason for such behavior is pain and fear of more pain.

He typically enjoys a network of friends whom were like-minded in many ways, and he enjoyed going to movies and hanging out with them when he had free time. Living in a co-ed dorm, it's easy to blend in as a student, and select what you want to do with free time, and with whom.

He is fortunate to find a few mutually appreciated 'friends with benefits' arrangements. He is still a friend with these ladies, and enjoys the mutual support and emotional intimacy the relationships offer.

Sometimes he misses the dorm life

and the mundane simplicity, drama and the convenience of it all. The dorm with a cafeteria and amenities nearby, is a casual, simple lifestyle. The relentless intensity,and demands of the residency training makes it difficult to have any type of personal or social relationship. Even if he has time, so many of the ladies seem to be incompatible to him; "It's not worth the effort to get involved," he tells himself. He has to wonder if it's the degree or himself that interests them. He has to admit to himself that others do not share his values or sense of fairness.

The rigors of medical education and training presents challenges to even established, committed relationships. Nearly all of the medical students whom are married when school starts are divorced by the time graduation occurs or in year one post graduate. As Henry had said, "There's no safe passage once you get accepted and enter the medical education process."

Due to the high, intense volume of information, the fast pace and demeanor of the program there is little room for normalcy. Ironically, one has to fully immerse themselves into the program to stay afloat in it. The isolation seems to be by design; keep you scared, tired, malnourished, and overwhelmed in order to mold your mind and behavior.

Meanwhile, his peers do not seem to notice. Reggie knows there is an indoctrination occurring slowly, but surely. He is glad that his parent's frequent mindset of a dubious and discerning nature are part of him.

From day one of the medical education there has been fear poured over him and others. The fear of being sued for malpractice is mentioned frequently. The fear of not knowing pertinent or relevant information and then getting sued for mistakes. It's a strange world and the selfish reactions of his peers betrays the fear that permeates them.

There is a game played whereas students they are put on a pedestal for being selected over others. Sometimes due to their family's political connections or due to policy changes that require quotas to be filled with gender, race or socioeconomic status. Ostensibly, selected due to their intelligence, but more often than not they are reminded of what they don't know. The name of the game is control in many areas; certainly in medical training. Admission is often acquired and not earned as high g.p.a. and Mcat scores do not gain admission.

The power the educational process has over them with just fear and subtle intimidation is great. It is a devious, integrated part of the training; keep student doctors tired, hungry and scared and you can shape them more easily.

The faculty admits that ninety percent of what they present is useless or inaccurate information, ten percent might be on a board exam or class exam and; less than one percent is useful, and relevant to the practice of medicine. Discerning which is the superfluous ninety-nine percent and which is the useful one percent is the name of that testing game.

Some of the faculty laugh and say, "Half of what we teach is obsolete or inaccurate, but which half is unknown."

What is certainly pushed is the reactive practice of pharmacology. This is to the exclusion of any other methods of treating diseases. Easily,the biggest mindset adjustment he has had to make is that health is **not** promoted. However, diseases and pathology are. It is a malignant, and dehumanizing, albeit profitable business model. It creates more business by standards of care to practice theory based medicine. "This is more like vocational school," he intuitively realizes during a rare moment of clarity.

The fear in the classrooms is palpable. It is like walking into a putrid fog of negativity. Even more so on exam days. He makes it a point to stay away until he absolutely has to go into the classroom on those days. Reggie notices the faculty talks about the need for compassion in the profession, but does not demonstrate it. Not while in their day to day activities or in their often inept teaching styles.

He learns quickly that medicine should actually be spelled m-*e*-*g*-*o*-d-i-c-i-n-e; as there is certainly ego in medicine; and some of the players certainly perceive themselves as god. The common self aggrandizement seems to be over the top for so many of the physicians and medical students. Their natural arrogance is amplified; jerks become bigger jerks!

He recalls a time when a fellow student used as a demonstrative prop pushes back. The student, often picked for demonstrations, discretely and tactfully asks the professor to use someone else as it is distracting them.

Instead of respecting the student's wishes as he agrees to the request during their conversation. The next day, instructor informs the class of the student's request not to be used for demonstrations, but he is going to use him anyway.

The instructors are either really good or really poor at teaching the course's content. The pace and volume of material presented is copious. If you fall behind there is no catching up. Generally, there is no safe passage upon admittance; unless someone is going to bat for you to influence the decision makers.

Reginald has to rely upon his attentiveness in class and his innate ability to recall, as there is very little time that can be used after the course work was complete for a given day.

The students are still competitive even in medical school they fought tooth and nail to get into. It is not unusual to find mandatory or helpful resources not where they are supposed to be in the library. Instead they are moved, and hidden by cliques of students. They know the location, but others do not. If they can get an advantage they do. As they are now competing for post-graduate training residency spots.

Reginald is surprised how self-centered his peers are. Often they come from privilege and often have never had to work for anything. They seem to be out of touch with how others live day to day. This impairs their ability to develop empathy let alone be empathic. Their education is being paid by family wealth, and they complete their education without the enslavement of debt obligations. He recalls the analogy Henry describes, "We are born riding a horse and saddle, but some of the saddle bags have more rocks than others; and some of the horses are pulling a load as well; it makes it difficult to move forward."

His wisdom is evident, and does not fall on deaf ears with Reginald. His innate curiosity, intelligence, and enthusiasm is conducive to learning, but not the insidious indoctrination.

"How can they relate to hardships of others, when they have no practical life experience that they can use to relate to others?"

He ponders as he watches the haughty attitudes in their encounters. At a personal values level he finds those attitudes repugnant. The individuals harboring those attitudes he notices are incredibly naive and out of touch. He finds it difficult to relate to them, and is glad that his encounters with them are polite and superficial in the day to day encounters.

He is middle class himself, as both parents work to obtain the 'American Dream' even if it means living pay check to pay check at times to pay more on the mortgage and automobile loans and a vacation every year.

He acquires a solid work ethic and an idea of how many in society exists economically. Many typically live one or two missed paychecks from bankruptcy. He is raised to display manners and courtesy as well as compassion. He soon discovers these are not automatic human qualities. He rarely sees these values manifest in his medical peers. The peer students are self-absorbed, contrived, and eager to get the degree, title, and perks that accompany the physician's role and position. Reggie recalls a student say he doesn't care what kind of doctor he becomes, but he's interested in the, "Power, prestige, pussy and money," accompanying the degree.

Reginald does not hear many talk about the caring part of the profession or the role to help people find health. All in all, it is incompatible with his gentle nature.

He is surprised by the amount of alcohol and recreational drug use by his peers. He witnesses first hand actual drug use or the indiscreet paraphernalia associated with use. The rolling papers, the bongs, the mortal and pestle for crushing up the stimulants. However, unless there happens to be an arrest associated with the use, a blind eye is turned to it. As long as students keep their grades in the passing zone, all is assumed to be well. At faculty and student functions he notices the large quantities of alcohol available, and they can certainly put it away. He understands some of their denial and recognition of it as a problem. The prolific substance abuse is a merely a symptom of problems at the individual and institutional's core psyche levels. This practice is not uncommon, but not disparaged either.

Needless to say, with the lack of camaraderie, Reginald feels isolated during the medical school experience. He often feels like quitting, but recalls Henry's wisdom to 'keep your eyes on the prize.'

His friend and mentor, Henry, cautions him that even upon acceptance in medical school, that likely there are some students arbitrarily removed. Henry is neutral about Reginald's career aspirations, but reiterates the need to follow his interests.

Reggie figures out some of the game quickly. At times he feels like a frog in a pot of water heating up slowly. He realizes what Henry means when he says, "Be careful and beware of how much of the profession's cool-aid; not just medicine, but nearly every profession you swallow...it's better to swish and spit it out when no one is looking; otherwise you give them your mind, body, and soul."

The further he gets into the educational 'program' whether it is in the classroom coursework or clerkships in hospitals or clinics; the more that concept becomes clear. He understands what his mentor means. He realizes its a closed system that does not like or tolerate anything other than its own paradigm.

He also realizes how little autonomy the physicians actually have within their chosen profession. The standards of care are developed by the pharmaceutical companies, and you deviate from them at your own peril.

He often hears attending physicians refer to it as 'cookbook medicine' with a degree of resignation and contempt at times. True to their training and indoctrination, they become sheep. They simply accept it as inevitable, shrug their shoulders, complain and comply. Fatalism is a symptom of a fearful, closed mind and a battered soul.

Even though the pharmaceutical companies do not directly pay their salaries; physicians are their unpaid, employees. The pharmaceutical companies are the hidden hand behind much of the policy, practice and delivery of contemporary healthcare.

The gullible physician is merely a

pawn in the scheme, not to produce better health, but to increase profits for the health care industry. With traditional health insurance plans replaced by managed health care organizations with the name of insurance companies; the public is duped as big business and pharmaceutical companies influence national legislative policy and create a business model and a disease management industry. Profit is the primary motive, not health.

They become unregulated, and unable to be touched by the various state insurance commissioners or anyone else. There is a reason their business models became HMO, PPO, Managed Care, because they are no longer insurance companies. For the most part, unregulated, they change the practice of medicine from a compassion based healing art to big business as usual. This is a far cry from creating health and promoting the common good and human evolution.

The vernacular of the profession

changes. For example, referring to their patients, 'customers,' or 'consumers' or the disparaging 'frequent flyer'. Another mind fuck occurs by calling increasing profits; 'cost-cutting'. These reflect the changes and the ironic dehumanization. Henry advises him of some of these observations and helps Reggie pick up on the subtleties. The astute Reggie picks up on this game. Even though his peers and physicians, preoccupied with being fearful, thinking of themselves, and concerned about paying the debt they are acquiring do not see it happening.

Reggie keeps his eyes on the prize. His motives for becoming a physician are altruistic. He wants to help people find and maintain health. His motive provides him some measure of comfort and strength, but it's still hard to get out of bed.

Reggie takes a few slow deep breathes and hold them before releasing them in an effort to energize himself.

Without trying to resist the fatigue, he nods off for a few moments sitting upright. Immediately starting to dream in the hypnogogic state he is between being awake and, being asleep. In the vision he sees a woman walking toward him. The auburn haired lady with jeans and a t-shirt and big framed glasses smiles and says, "I don't belong here." This awakens him and he stands to prevent another episode of dozing off

The modest salary of a resident physician enables him to live in a less than affluent; some might call it a sketchy area; others a ghetto. Every morning he leaves his humble abode expecting to find his car broken into. He is always relieved when it is not. He make sure there are no coins, shiny objects, food, clothing or electronics left in his car lest it tempt someone to break in and take it.

This is not a good area to live, so an unwanted guest is within the realm of possibility. The image awakens him, as he did not know her or recognize her. He raises himself, sitting upright in the bed with his heart beating rapidly. He looks around the dimly lit room to reorient himself and realize he is alone. "Now, I need to get up," he thinks. "I wonder what that dream is about."

He rolls over to his right and allows his long legs to descend. Long gone are the days of leaping out of bed excited about the upcoming events of the day. His bare feet on the ancient, fading beige, shag carpet is likely as old as the original construction. It feels dusty and worn beneath his bare feet. He regrets not having socks to prevent the history of the carpet from sticking on his feet. The carpet has seen better days, he walks quickly to move across it hoping a nasty fungus does not stick to his sole.

He opts for a cold shower. Henry suggests he try them a few years ago and he still follows the suggestion of his mentor. He likes it, because the cold shower stimulates the immune system, and increases alertness, and pulls in prana from the environment. Reggie adapts readily to good advice and incorporates into his life; this is a sign of real intelligence.

For Reggie, it is an effort to help him not only awaken, but also to feel something. The water is so cold that it feels like needles upon his scalp. He feels the cold water hit and cascade off his scalp.

He remembers to take a deep breath as he tilts his head back, the cold water feels refreshing on his face. He relaxes his facial muscles to resist the reflex urge to tense them. "This feels good," he smiles as he puts some thick, fragrant shampoo in the palm of his right hand to suds up his hair.

It is not easy with cold water, but he manages to massage the soap into his hair and scalp. He likes the feel of the cooler water on him as it reminds him he can still feel something at a visceral and etheric level.

The water and shampoo mixture feels warm as it flows down his legs. "I must be hot," he muses as he notices the temperature difference of water hitting him and rolling off of him. He relaxes his bladder and allows his body to release the overnight accumulation of urine. He raises his arms to get the cold liquid over the lateral sides of his body. Now the water feels like an elixir as he allows the spray to cover him completely. He finally feels alert, alive and reasonably refreshed.

He hears his alarm go off again, but he is on top of his game; for the moment. His short hair is easily wiped dry with a thick towel. He smears the conditioner on his neck and cheeks to assist the act of shaving the facial hair that occurs daily. The tooth brush covers every exposed area of his teeth and the flossing is so second nature he does not require a mirror to assist him in the health promoting daily task.

He grabs his long white coat which hangs from the top corner of the closet door. The pockets are still full of notes he's taken and the small clinician's manual he uses to determine everything from mean arterial pressure, to flow rates for I.V. saline drips. He has come to rely on it less, but likes having it close at hand. His stethoscope is coiled smoothly and compactly in the other large pocket. It will remain there until he gets into the hospital, whereupon he'll drape it over his shoulders and around his neck. Nothing projects the image of a doctor like a stethoscope and a long white coat.

The long white coat is a welcome addition instead of the short white coat that hangs on the shoulders of medical students; the swagger is not there with the short white coat. The profession has many integrated ways of keeping the neophytes in their place.

The profession's educational and

training process is abusive mentally and physically. The first flaw is the competitive nature; it's often not a matter of excellent g.p.a.'s or MCAT score, but connections or quotas that provide the entrance. Who you know, or who you owe is alive and well.

Another flaw inherent, in the process, is established doctors want the new doctors to have it as brutal as they had it. Many of them being so caught up in getting into medical school starting in their teens and twenties their emotional development got stuck somewhere in late adolescence or early adulthood. Since stress interferes with the connection of the frontal lobes; their adult features don't match the immature, and often narcissistic mindsets they carry with them. This is not by accident; it is essentially a highfalutin vocational school; not a place to encourage healing and find health.

Masquerading as mature, adults as

well as caring physicians they shape the naive, young minds which are the future of medicine. This self perpetuating cycle with few physicians seeing the bull-shit and challenging or improving the situation or circumstances.

Reggie is not the typical out of the frying pan into the fire medical student becoming a physician. He has a work ethic, but lacks the sense of entitlement and self aggrandizement that he frequently sees. He is still a nice guy despite being put through the wringer of the education also known programming process.

He finds employment at an engineering firm for two years upon completing his degree. He finds the work to be interesting and engaging at times, but most of the time it is boring and generally unfulfilling. The salary is respectable, but he desires to be challenged and the engineering position is underwhelming. Henry has a standing offer to hire him at his lab anytime he wants and put his degree to pursuing innovative, creative work.

He is considering Henry's offer, but heeds the medical calling after helping a non-responsive employee at a job site. The encounter surprisingly is not awkward or uncomfortable to him. He calmly checks to make sure the middle-aged, obese gentleman was breathing, found a pulse and chatting with him while awaiting the EMT's arrival.

He knew at that moment that he could become a physician. Recalling his mentor and friend, Henry's suggestion to follow his interest, he completes the MCAT and applies to schools that appeals to him location wise.

He prefers warmer climes and let that guide him. He stays away from the northern states and applies locally as well. Gaining acceptance to the school is the easiest part; and that says a lot.

He's not hung up on the prestige and superficial trappings. He soon arrives at an insight through casual observation that they're referred to as trappings, because they seem to hold people hostage. Materialism continues to trump spiritualism for many individuals at the expense of their humanity.

Appearances, and maintaining them seem to be superfluous and a waste of time and energy. He finds random thoughts 'coming' to him such as part of the world's problem is people working for money rather than working to evolve, and improve the world. Feeling at times like square in a worlds of circles. He wants to believe everyone thinks like he does, but instead he is finding many do not think much at all. The idea of an original thought might be the most original thought they create. He sees many just being creatures of habit, and influenced by the long term, insidious institutional indoctrination that begins upon birth. A relatively few number of people and institutions shape our thinking, thoughts, and point of view

It is much easier to go along, and get along, do not think critically, and to look out for number one. It's a habit that is so pervasive it seems to be a normal cathexis.

Chapter Two

Journal entry:

 I was finally treated like a human being for a few
minutes today. I actually had an attending stand up for
me! It's incredible that something that should be so
ordinary, everyday, and benign is the exception and not
the rule. It feels good to have the long coat of
physician and no longer have to wear the short coat of
the student. I have no qualms about parking in the
Doctors Only spaces even with my less than immaculate
ride. My car is a metaphor for my life right now. It
began new, and fresh, but is now unkempt, neglected, and
abused; reduced to a mere, basic transportation; a tool,
and in desperate need of TLC and maintenance. Of course,
I have no spare time to perform or money to take care
of it. I don't mind being a physician in training, but these
attending physicians are not god. And after going into
the bathroom after them; their shit does stink! I hope I
have better hygiene than Doctor Morton; he is so gross! I
am getting my fill of the bullshit. I actually felt a surge
of anger go through me today...Thank God, I caught
myself going to a very unfamiliar, but dark place for a
moment before I got myself back on track...This is not
me....Where's the compassion? Where's the love? How can
this situation be right?

Morning Rounds

Reggie is definitely not by any stretch, a pretentious individual, and is very humble. However, he does not hesitate to park his modest sedan in spaces clearly marked 'Doctors Only'. Like the long, white coat; that parking space is earned. His car needs new tires, a tune up, and the squeaking from the front reminds him it needs new brakes. The air conditioner only blowing cool air needs service. On the outside it's dull silver paint in need of a wash and wax rolls indignantly to a squeaking stop.

It enters the spot complete with several months accumulation of dried, dead bugs plastered on the grill, headlights, hood, and dirty windshield boldly eases into the parking spot reserved for 'doctors only'. The audible squeaking of the worn, brake linings announce his arrival to no one in particular; it nestles in the spot.

Reggie cannot hear the squeak

thanks to the CD blaring his favorite heavy metal tune. He feels pumped thanks to the guitar rifts, and garbled lyrics.

Grabbing his crumpled, white coat, which is usually hastily thrown in as a silent passenger. Exiting the car and gracefully putting the white coat over his shoulder and guides his arms through the long sleeves far from the freshly starched appearance they had a few weeks ago fresh from the cleaning service.

The sun is still low in the eastern sky. It is still dark as puts on his white coat which is conspicuous in low light. He pats his pockets to make sure he has what he needs to complete the morning rounds. The shiny, deep black, ballpoint ink designer pens are in the breast pocket, the stethoscope coiled in his right pocket. The internal medicine manuals he will need to reference are in his left with dog-eared pages, and sticky notes added are making it thicker now than original neat, compact size.

He feels the soft, cotton, light

scrub bottoms he is wearing. With the surgery rotation, a different dress code is tolerated. "All right! No shirt and tie today," he walks briskly and deliberately toward the entrance.

His sneakers stride confidently along the smooth pavement; he brings on a swag for a few strides and then leaves it in the parking lot. The strut, and swag is unofficially reserved for the attending physicians once you're in the hospital. A cocky resident is an easy target for additional bull-shit extra pimping, and scut work.

This is the start of a dynamic day. He discretely listens to the murmur of the emergency department doctors and staff as he walks through the doors that smoothly automatically open for anyone approaching.

From what he can gather as he slows down ostensibly to get a cup of the always brewed coffee, but to eavesdrop and hear of a couple of patients that died overnight. Immediately recognizing some of the patients names as the elderly, 'frequent flyers'. They are called that because they seem to always be in the hospital; their admissions blend together.

"Huh," he muses, "They are all Doctor Morton's patients, at the rate he is losing his current admissions he may not need coverage when he takes his vacation after all."

Doctor Morton is an institution within the hospital and has practiced medicine for forty years starting with his residency at the same hospital. With his stoop posture, and gray, receding hairline, dark spots on his skin, he looks older than his sixty-eight years. He reeks of stale cigarettes and has the blue color of the mentholyptus flavored cough drops, which he uses in an effort to reduce his smoking habit visible on the corner of his mouth.

He has a middle age paunch and thin, bony shoulders as he plods along, he often wears a scowl; which keeps individuals at distance. He is aloof at times, cordial at others. This gives him the unpredictability that keeps their encounters at a distance. For years, the nurses, staff and his patients constantly complain about his hygiene, condescending demeanor and rudeness.

However, he is not the only doctor like that. The hospital's administration protects their physicians as well as their bottom line. The appointed upper level administrators do not look at him or his role personally, but as a money maker.

As long as they produce money; they and their quirks are tolerated, and turning a blind eye and a deaf ear is the norm and the de facto method of doing business. Money is always in the equation, medical care is a big business; not a healing profession.

Doctor Morton wears plaid, loud, colorful polyester slacks he's had for so long they become fashionable again. Sometimes you can see the small, holes burned into the fabric by the stray ash of a long forgotten cigarette. If he were standing alone on a busy street corner, with his stooped appearance, old polyester attire, and nicotine stained fingers he might appear to be a down on their luck homeless man.

He shuffles by Reggie, who does not time his inhaled breath properly. As a result he caught a whiff of the stale, acrid cigarette odor that emanates from the older doctor. "Hello, young Doctor Washington," he exhales as the mixture of stale cigarettes and black coffee pummels Reggie. As a reflex, he catches himself leaning back to escape the confines of the encounter. "Did you read that article on managing glucose levels in patients with fragile diabetes that I left in your mailbox?"

"Yes, I did," Reggie replies quickly and then he holds his breath to avoid the toxic breath from the lungs of Doctor Morton. He actually read that article on his own months before Doctor

Morton left him a copy.

"So what do you think?" Doctor Morton asks while rubbing the back of his hairy hand across the bridge of his nose; his unibrow conspicuous.

"Here comes the pimping," Reggie thinks as he quickly recalls some salient points of the article. "Well, tighter controls of glucose levels are desirable," he says as he gauges the nonverbal responses of the attending physician and realizes he is not impressed; so he quickly continues, "The hemoglobin A1C number, not their self reporting, is the best test to see if patient is compliant with tighter controls."

Reggie's rapid response to his question catches Doctor Morton off guard as it is obvious Reggie has perused at the article. "Well," he stammers for a moment and recovers to ask, "And how do patients become compliant?"

"The literatures points out that with education, family and physician's support and positive feedback," Reggie responds quickly. "Yes, and what is the biggest barrier to compliance?" Doctor Morton, surprised by the reply, elevates his eyebrow.

"If financial barriers are removed, it is more than likely due to the patient's psychodynamic, interpersonal or intra-personal metrics." His swift replies makes Doctor Morton feel uncomfortable, but he is also impressed as well nodding his head and folding his arms, he seems at a loss.

"Well, yes," he replies as he turns to shuffle away muttering something about doing a dictation.

"Nice...nice job Reggie," He hears a soft hand clap from across the hall.

"Good morning, Doctor Kutnem," Reggie replies recognizing the voice of the surgeon that he wishes he had been assigned to mentor him on the surgical rotation.

Raising his foot he exclaims, "I'm glad I wore my boots after hearing that monologue you gave to Doctor Morton. Hell, you even had me believing it." Laughter punctuates his sentence.

"Hey, what I said was the truth wasn't it?" he respectfully asks.

"Yes, and even if it wasn't true, the way you delivered it with such confidence and lack of hesitancy. It would have got by even the most asinine attending!"

"You think so?"

"Absolutely, remember that the confidence projected in how you say something is just as important as what you say."

"Thanks for the sage wisdom, Doctor Kutnem. I appreciate it"

"You just did it again...are you full of shit or what?"

"Uh, uh no Doctor Kutnem, I really mean it, I really appreciate-"

Doctor Kutnem's burst of belly laughter interrupts Reggie's sentence, "See what I mean," he says with a playful grin betraying the humor; "You residents can be so serious all of the time."

"Yeah, I got it..." Reggie is not sure whether to let his guard down or remain vigilant.

Doctor Kutnem is not the typical surgeon. He is skilled, competent, meticulous and conscientious, but not overbearing, or arrogant. All of them have to be skilled technicians and pay really high liability insurance rates, but they play a role that is not easy.

As a surgeon, he is compassionate, mindful and believes that patients can still hear conversations even if they are unconscious. This belief and practice is not shared by many of his peers.

He tactfully encourages operation room staff to be mindful of what they say, even in jest while assisting an operation. As a result, procedures flow smoothly and his patients generally have a swift and uneventful recovery. He speaks directly to the unconscious patient at times, and plays classical music in the cold, sterile background before and while the procedure is occurring. Staff try hard to get on his support team.

"How is your training coming along?" He asks with sincerity and not the usual contrived fishing question. He asks because it is an appropriate question to ask.

Reggie is taken aback by the question, and leans back in a startled response, but composes himself. "I'm just so tired, and I wonder if I can ever do anything right."

Doctor Kutnem shakes his head, and leans forward,"Sounds like the same old bullshit. Unfortunately, the crude barbaric ways physicians are trained can create a monster at worst or a machine at best."

Looking at Reggie to gauge his reaction, he continues, "As you've likely noticed many of the attendings lack people skills; and even worse, they don't even realize it. They may have intellectual compassion and empathy if you are lucky, but they cannot do it naturally or authentically."

"Yeah, yeah!" Reggie replies nods slowly."So,it's not my imagination!"

Doctor Kutnem gives Reggie a soft gaze, and touches him on his sleeve, "No, it's just a deeply flawed, but equally deeply entrenched system."

"Thank you Doctor, Need to hear that from outside my own head!"

Journal entry:

It is so nice to have someone actually ask about my well-being like Doctor Kutnem did today; not in a contrived, polite banter sort of way, but sincerely wanting to know about what's going on with me...he is a great human being, and a great physician...I add him to my positive mentor list...I like what I see...I want to be calm, and competent like him someday...competent, compassionate, and not arrogant, and self-centered...He is more evolved than any physician I've met...even though he does not identify with any religious faith; he is more of a Christian than those constantly proselytizing their faith with their abundant verbiage...Doctor Morton is a walking seminar on how not to be...he is self-centered, a bully, and an ass-hole...It's bitter sweet to have a nice encounter, because it's a reminder that it is that bad at times. I got pimped by Doctor Morton today, and nailed it! I could only speak the party line, and could not go into alternative interventions such as supplementation and dietary changes, because it is not acceptable, and I would be seen as less than competent.

Reggie releases an audible sigh and allows his shoulders to descend, "It is what it is." he covers his mouth.

"So, it's still a lot of bull-shit, huh?" He replies with truthful empathy and eye contact to gauge Reggie's response.

"Yeah," he replies perking up, and an errant tear forms on the corner of his right eye. For the first time in a long time, Reggie actually felt that someone has empathy not by contrived statements or cliches, but by actually relating to him.

For better or worse, he has found the medical training at all levels continues to be fraught with ego, arrogance and aggrandizement and lack of compassion that provides a lack of any support in the medical training.

"You know Reggie," standing, he leads him into a private, secluded room usually reserved for dictation and private conferences, "Nearly every part of the medical system is bull-shit, and knowing that makes the practice of medicine more tolerable." Touching his index finger to his chin and looking away for a moment in a pause before continuing, "The first step to problem solving is identifying the problem, and protecting yourself."

Reggie nods and rubs his chin and cheeks with his hands. He does this subconsciously as an effort to cope with the intense emotion of the moment.

"This is not a noble profession and certainly not one that takes the best people to become physicians. Whether you and I want to believe it or not, we are to one degree or another, basically unpaid, extended employees of the pharmaceutical industry and health care coverage providers."

"You mean insurance companies?" Reggie asks to clarify.

"There are no insurance companies anymore, they have been replaced by largely unregulated managed care, HMO's, PPO's and other such nonsense."

"Really?" Reggie replies as his jaw spontaneously goes slack.

"Yes, thanks to the lobbyist's influence on our state and federal legislators we have by proxy. And by trusting our hands to the inept professional organization to be watchdogs, we allow the foxes to take over the henhouse."

"How could that happen?" Reggie articulates.

"Complacency, and as you will discover if you have not already; rust never sleeps. We, as professionals, forget that as there are more regulations, you have to sacrifice autonomy, and ability to innovate."

"That's not good to hear." Reggie replies with resignation in his voice.

Nodding, Doctor Kutnem replies, "This did not happen overnight or in a single decision. The profession has unfortunately surrendered its autonomy incrementally. They can't do much to surgeons whom practice limited medicine, but they can control others, and now the professionals and the patients have to endure the consequences."

"What are the consequences?" Reggie asks making sure he is on the same page.

"Well, for starters, the classic divide and conquer paradigm. What begins as a seemingly benevolent, sensible, and inconspicuous profession can change. It becomes a profit driven, disease management profession. It creates an adversarial relationship, between the profession and the patients, and the often naive, or ignorant healthcare professionals."

"What do you mean?" Reggie asks realizing that he does not know everything; he's comfortable with that.

65

"For instance, if a patient is readmitted within thirty days of discharge for a previously treated diagnosis; the hospital has to return any reimbursement and then correct the problem at their own expense."

"No way!" Reggie shakes his head incredulously, "But what if the patient is noncompliant, and does not follow discharge plans? What are we supposed to do hold their hand?"

"I see you are understanding what I mean?" Doctor Kutnem smiles as he sees that Reggie is getting the jest of the conversation.

"Yeah...yeah and if they stop taking the medicine or never get the prescription filled to begin with, for whatever reason, the responsibility is still on us,the physician." Reggie feels good being able to refer to himself with the 'p' word.

"Yes,the physician's responsibility to the patient is greater than their responsibility to us."

"That's messed up!"

"Tell me about it, inevitably it makes the doctor patient interaction an adversarial encounter versus a co-creative encounter with the patient taking their share of responsibility for their care and health; many patients are content to put their lives and health in someone else's hands."

"How did it get to this point?" Reggie asks with his mind still reeling.

"We trust others that we appoint or elect to represent us in positions of power and influence to look out for our best interests; and apparently, they didn't do that; so here we are."

"Can this be fixed?" Reggie asks furrowing his brow. His breathing has become shallow and more rapid as his heart responds to the exasperation and anger of adrenaline; he feels warm.

Doctor Kutnem grimaces, takes a deep breath and looks toward the ceiling before answering, "Not likely, we have surrendered so much to others who have their own interests at heart over the profession, they are not likely to give up the ground they've acquired; possession is indeed nine-tenths. And don't get me started on the whole mandatory vaccination requirement. Anything mandatory is a different level of coercion altogether "

Reggie sits quietly as all of these revelations sink into his discernment thinking processes. "What you've described is surreal. Like a black and white Twilight Zone episode." He says with the revelations hitting his discernment buttons and resonating to his truth centers.

"Did they cover any of this in your course work in undergrad or medical school?" This is a rhetorical question he asks to calm himself.

"Not at all," Reggie replies as he sees Doctor Kutnem's furrowed brow. To cut the tension he adds, "Have you seen Henry lately?"

"No," he replies, "But I'm having

dinner with him and Kris this weekend; I'll tell him you asked about him." He and Reggie glance up and see a scowling Doctor Ashley peering through the rectangular window. Doctor Ashley opens the door without knocking and enters and glares intensely at Reggie.

Reggie feels a surge of anger and is prepared to ask him 'what the fuck is your problem', but before he can escalate Doctor Kutnem intervenes.

"Doctor Ashley," Doctor Kutnem greets him by standing as he walks in, "I was just inviting Doctor Washington to assist me with a procedure this afternoon, that is if you can cut him loose from your clinic."

Doctor Ashley is caught off guard by the forwardness of Doctor Kutnem. "Uh, sure...not much is going on at the clinic, and I know you have his education and training in mind."

"Certainly, and an umbilical hernia repair is always instructional; thank you for allowing him to assist me." The appropriateness and professionalism exhibited by Doctor Kutnem is certainly appreciated by Reggie. He suspects that many simply tolerate the overbearing, narcissism of Doctor Ashley.

"Now, don't give him a hard time, because I corralled him on his way to making rounds; this is still a teaching hospital." Doctor Kutnem says while giving Doctor Ashley an intense glare, "Also, Doctor Washington is my friend."

For a brief, awkward moment, Reggie notices a split second expression of fear on the Doctor Ashley's face. He feels safe for an instant which is unusual in a training program that uses fear to control and motivate their indentured servants. He wants to cheer, but he maintains his poise and graciously thanks Doctor Kutnem for the invitation, and verifies the when and where of the afternoon procedure.

Reggie walks behind Doctor Ashley who is going down the long corridor of off-white tiles. Reggie knows the attending physicians are at the lead, followed by residents, interns and medical students. It makes sense as the more experienced lead, and the less experienced follow.

There is a hierarchy and although it is an unwritten rule; it is generally understood as a custom. "Doctor Kutnem schools Doctor Ashley," Reggie thinks as a flash smile passes quickly across his demeanor, "I hope he doesn't give me a payback for this."

He is pleasantly distracted as the petite, brunette approaches. She makes eye contact and smiles at Reggie. He can't help, but smile back at her. Her blue eyes sparkle as she smiles. She is discrete and professional in her role. Her sincere and sweet demeanor was something that Reggie noticed when they met and were mutually attracted. It took only a few hours together to click.

As she passes he glances over to see her also glance back, and smile at him. She puts her fist with thumb up and little finger out next to her ear and mouths the words, "Call me." She is carrying her large purse and is likely leaving her shift. She is one of the PRN LPNs that make his shifts more rewarding.

Rocio is bright, has a great sense of humor and amazing charisma. Blue eyes aren't common on a Latina, but are certainly appreciated by Reggie. He is thankful to have had the occasion to stare into the deep blue pools that seem to go on forever.

She can make Reggie's day when she finds the time and place to get physically and emotionally close. During her breaks and when things are in synch she has makes time in the call room pleasantly pass as she and Reggie find solace and a burst of companionship in their infrequent exchanges of intimate conversation and touch. She even provides the condoms for their brief, intense interludes that become physical.

He really likes her, and she likes

him, but the attending can currently provide a better situation for her. She hasn't told Reggie this, but he gets it,and is okay with the arrangement.

It's not practical to meet outside of work, so they continue their amorous dance of discretionary contact and mutual admiration. Reggie has no time or desire for another relationship, and he is fine with that. Residency is a challenging emotional and physical affair by itself.

A smile creases his face as reminisces,"Why don't you get some coffee, while I round," Reggie suggests as they walk in step, "You've only got couple of patients here."

"That'll be fine, meet me in the lounge and present the patients." Doctor Ashley comments peering over the top of his reading glasses.

"Okay, I'll be there as soon as I finish rounding the adult floor...it shouldn't take long."

Reggie figures out quickly that

Doctor Asher is picky about his patients he chooses to perform surgery. He does not take any case that might be risky.

He is like many general surgeons, his bread and butter consists of the constant flow of uncomplicated cholecystectomies,hysterectomies, hernioplastys, and appendectomies. He is quick to start them on narcotics with a fever reducer while they are in post-op. He brags about the lack of fever his patients have as if he is the most skilled surgeon available. He declines the tougher or complicated cases; that practice likely improves everyone's outcome.

Doctor Kutnem typically takes the more challenging cases, and performs them with great skill and relative ease. He is meticulous and competent, and more collegial than Doctor Asher.

Doctor Kutnem is well liked and respected by the OR crew. They are professionals in their own right, and often undervalued, and unappreciated by the attending physicians. However, when Doctor Kutnem is on the schedule, they clamor to be able to assist him. Reggie is very excited to assist him later in the day.

As Reggie picks up the patient's records he looks at the nursing reports. "Temperature is normal, no complaints of pain, no elevated blood pressure," he thinks. He washes his hands, and moves the gown to look at the surgical site.

His systematic thinking takes over as he takes in the patient's presentation. Some of the training is good, logical, and health promoting. There is no warmth, no inflammation, no tenderness upon palpation. All of these observed findings are good signs that the post-op patient is avoiding complications.

"You have warm, soft hands," the patient comments, "By the way, thanks for washing your hands before touching me. I really appreciate it."

"You're welcome," he replies.

"Doesn't every healthcare professional wash their hands before they touch you?"

"No! Sometimes I have to remind them; and believe me; having to do that is so annoying, and disturbing at many levels."

"That is disturbing," Reggie replies with contempt trailing the words and his head nodding.

"Did Doctor Asher say when I can get out of here?'

"I knew you would ask me that." He comments and after a sigh; continues. "As you have figured out; residents don't get to control the discharge date. We only assist in managing your case until then."

"So you can't help me get out of here as soon as this morning?"

"Well, you know Doctor Ashley will be the one ordering a discharge," Reggie replies. "Have you had a BM?" He asks using the hospital vernacular for a bowel movement.

"No, but I'm eating. That should help with the bowel movement."

Reggie smiles and nods as he pats his arm, "You're correct, that's a start, that's good. Are you able to get up and walk around?"

"I can get up, but haven't walked outside the room. I'd like to move around more if I can."

"Sure, if you can; do it. Walking around, especially outside the room will help your bowels move," Reggie nods. "Also, it's good your temperature is normal, and you are able to get up, your appetite is back; the only thing really keeping you here is a lack of a BM."

"Doc, can you get me something for that? I really want to get out of here; no offense, but I hate hospitals."

Reggie nods, "I hear you, but protocols are protocols. Lets try the hot coffee with your breakfast. If you drink it before eating you'll get better results. Do that and after breakfast try walking around to see if that works before we go to the medicine chest. Perhaps you can have your wife bring some magnesium citrate that is can help expedite the process."

"That's over the counter?"

"Yes, and you need it anyway, as you know, the pain medicine can cause constipation. It appears you had your last dose last night; is your pain an issue?" Reggie asks hoping it does not open pandora's box as it is the fifth vital sign, but such a subjective question.

"Well, I'm tired, and a little sore."

"As well you should be." dropping to a knee, and keeping eye contact, he responds pragmatically, succinctly, but also compassionately as well. "It's called surgery, and you were stabbed with a scalpel, had a gall bladder cut off your liver. The bleeding detected is cauterized with intense heat, the gall bladder is then removed from a small approximately three centimeter opening.

Then, you are sewn together with a sharp needle and thick thread tearing through your thin skin. It is called surgery, but outside the hospital it would be called a felony assault and someone could go to prison for a while!"

A chuckle from the patient lets Reggie know he is listening, "So you're saying the soreness is normal?"

"Yes, and desirable as well. I would be gravely concerned if you aren't sore" Reggie likes to keep it real with honesty and plain talk that the patients can easily understand. Medical jargon can be a mask to cover its diminishing humanity.

"Okay, thank you Doctor."

"Any more questions before I go?" Reggie asks rhetorically

"Will Doctor Asher be around to see me?"

"Definitely, if you think of any questions, don't hesitate to ask him."

"Ask me what?" Doctor Ashley has entered the room as his overbearing nature could not allow him to wait a few minutes.

"Nice," Reggie thinks, "I want to get out of here."

"I'll finish rounds and catch up with you," Reggie is deliberately leaving the room to prevent being further detained by the overbearing surgeon.

Although, he is officially a Doctor and physician, he is still in training. Reggie is frustrated by attending physicians who want you to manage the cases, until you actually start managing them and then they do not the proactive behavior of physicians in training. Reggie is frustrated by the catch-22 situations. If you manage the case, whether by writing orders for consults, tests or medicines you cannot win. If you order a test or drug the attending physician overlooked or did not typically use; you are out of line even if it was a good idea or intervention. However, if you did not add any changes to the case you're out of line is well.

Teaching and mentoring is sadly a lost art for many of the attending physicians; and they hardly understand the what and why of what they're doing. They simply parrot what they have been told. No original thought, intelligence or creativity is encouraged.

Journal entry:

I am appalled by the lack of compassion and empathy of my peers in the residency program. They cannot get past themselves. If something does not directly impact them it is irrelevant. Yeah, they're young and immature, but so are the attending physicians who seem to be stuck in the mindset they had as twenty-something year old residents. I get so tired of the assholes who want to be a doctor with the prestige and pay, but see no need to develop and evolve. Humility is non existent, and they are so closed to stepping out of their comfort zone...I do not trust them either, but I have to be collegial with them, but I know that if they could they would use me as a stepping stone if it could elevate their status.

He finds himself early for the early morning resident's meeting. The conference room has some comfortable chairs and soft lighting; it seems apart from the rest of the hospital. Sitting quietly in the room, eyes closed, hands clasped, chin tucked and automatically taking some slow deep breaths.

He enjoys the solitude even as it is disrupted by the heavy steps and bleary, tired eyes of a peer, Roderick, who is finishing his first overnight shift. At that time, Reggie attempts to give him a heads up on what to expect, but the arrogant, and aloof Roderick dismisses his conversation and was not seeking a collegial encounter.

"I can't believe how incompetent the nurses are," Roderick blurts out with the veins on his neck and forehead protruding and nostrils flared. His trembling hands made into white knuckled fists. Reggie can sense the exhaustion, frustration and anger; it's very raw, and uncomfortable.

Reggie turns his head to the left, and leans his body to the right to acknowledge his presence. As Roderick escalates his rant; his eyes wide open.

"They call me over the stupidest, fucking things...or don't call me at all when they should! It is so fucking unbelievable!" As he enunciates his words, his face is beet red,and both of his external jugular veins are bulging prominently and his hands are trembling from anger and fatigue. Saliva drains from the corner of his mouth; his eyes are dull and red.

Nodding in silent acknowledgment Reggie replies, "It is what it is. Some of the nurses are savvy and others are still in the learning curve. Just like us." This is in contrast to the smug, silent, condescending, smirk that Roderick provided him two months earlier. "I had the same issues with them." Reggie says matter of factly to normalize the experience.

Reggie experienced what he later figured was hazing from them in retrospect when he did some night work. Roderick was void of empathy and compassion, but full of arrogance.

"Well, they should be more fucking
competent and professional!" Roderick
says spitting his anger out along with
the words; his knuckles are white.

Reggie nods and turns back around,
and resumes his previous position. "I
hear you," he reiterates hoping Roderick
shuts the fuck up. Roderick storms off
to pace the about the hall still
frustrated and angry. Reggie, is glad as
he takes a deep breath and closes his
eyes . It'll be a few minutes before he
has to be alert again.

"No need to get sucked into other
people's drama." He thinks as he drifts
off to sleep, awakening immediately a
few minutes later as others enter the
room. This is a skill he is continuing
to master, because he is so tired. In
two hours he is scheduled to be at the
family outpatient clinic again. He plans
on napping as long as possible before
traveling while too sleepy across town;
sleep and rest are at a premium.

<u>Journal Entry</u>:

I like, actually I enjoy, the time spent at the outpatient clinic. There is less micromanaging, and it's just you and the patient. Patients can be very entertaining without even trying. I had two patient encounters today that made me forget I was tired. The first encounter was a 53 year old male getting his blood pressure checked, and requesting a new prescription. He wanted an erectile dysfunction medicine to assist in, "Keeping my dick hard". I nod and speak to him about how erectile dysfunction could be a harbinger of bad news regarding the health of the cardiovascular system. He cut me off at that point, to clarify, "I don't have trouble getting an erection, but the pills help when I have a threesome." That statement caught me off guard, and my jaw likely dropped open. He replies, "I take it you haven't had a threesome before...they're not uncommon especially when you're a bartender." He said it so matter of factly, it's a safe bet it is a common occurrence in his world. I explain to him that the hypertension makes it too risky to prescribe those medications to him. I also explain to him that a prescription for that type of drug is a red flag for insurance underwriters of all types as they can surmise by medicine that he has cardiovascular issues or diabetic issues. He respectfully acknowledges understanding that, and asks, "How would they find out," if he didn't tell them. I explain that HIPAA is a data base, and that many have access to it. The medicines would be a red flag, and likely result in higher medical and life insurance coverage.

He thanks me for the education, and agrees to get his diastolic blood pressure lower. He is reluctant to use the prescription diuretics, and asks for alternatives. I explain he is likely deficient, and magnesium, and to take at least four hundred milligrams of magnesium citrate which is available over the counter, and to sip some apple cider vinegar until it tastes foul daily. That combination will regulate fluid, and the vinegar removes excess sodium which drives up the upper number of the blood pressure. He left feeling optimistic. It is nice to be able to help someone beyond handing them a prescription. The next even more curious patient encounter perks me up a bit more. It involves a female couple involved in a self described 'monogamous' relationship. The presenting complaint was fatigue, morning nausea, weight gain, and a missed menstrual period. Despite her insistence of no sexual intercourse with a man, I order a routine pregnancy test[and it tests positive. With that news, the patient is understandably shocked, but her partner has an expression of a cat that ate the canary. I explain its possible for a false positive to occur, but an OB-GYN referral to confirm it with a fetal Doppler. She is not happy, but agrees to the referral. As the distraught patient excuses herself, her partner stays behind. "Can I help you?" I ask not sure what to expect. She explains she leans more to the bisexual orientation rather than the pure gay female. She explains she had intercourse with a man who provided her a copious ejaculation earlier, and she did not have an opportunity to shower or douche before returning.

Because the partner did not like her friend; she did not tell her partner of this encounter, and they had sex after she arrived home that same evening. She explains there is no penetration with toys; however there might have been some finger penetration and digital stimulation. She said they engaged in tribbing, which by her description is another term for scissoring and grinding their vulvas. She inquires if it is possible that some of the semen could have gotten introduced to her partner at that time. I nod affirmatively, and watch as she quickly breaks out in a cold sweat, and turns pale approaching a panic attack.

    To break the tension, I make a comment about how a virgin pregnancy is apparently possible. She laughs as the pallor returns to her skin. "What should I tell her? Who is the father?" She asks. "Those questions are out of my areas of expertise," I tell her to not get too worried until the pregnancy is confirmed. I advise her to find a couples psychotherapist, and that the paternity determination, and responsibility sounds like a legal issue; which is definitely out of the scope of my license. This could be an interesting legal predicament, and precedent. It is good to have such an out of the ordinary mundane viral or allergy complaints that seem to keep the clinic busy. It is nice to have an out of the norm clinical experience that keeps my communication skills sharp. It is also nice to be respected by patients. The clinic resident's preceptor noticing the positive pregnancy test and seeing the distraught patient leave entered the room. Her response surprised me when she joined the meeting, and starts asking questions that seem to be more voyeuristic than necessary. She wants details, and specifics which seems to be for her personal benefit, and not related to the management of the case. I believe she was getting off on the situation. She stood unblinking, staring at the patient's partner, and soon develops a red rash on her neck. A weird reaction, and even the patient's partner was getting uncomfortable. I interrupt the awkward situation by reiterating the need to see what the situation actually is, not what it might be before moving forward. It surprises me how the attending physician is wanting to go in the weeds in a situation that could involve legal issues later. Her need to be a clinical voyeur is over the top. She is married with children, but she seems intrigued by the lesbian, and she appears to be flirting with the patient's partner. I hope I don't get any passive aggressive payback for stepping in and speaking up, but someone had to be the professional.

Chapter Three

Journal Entry: I wish I had more time for myself. I am getting tired of not having time for myself. I work, I sleep and do nothing for myself in between. My time is not my own, and the director of medical education is not sympathetic. They figure if they had to endure the post graduate education's bullshit so should anyone and everyone. They have no respect for your time. It is not easy to find the time and energy to mail bill payments or even get down time. They have no respect for your time at all...I don't even have time to develop any meaningful relationships or maintain the few I have.

Working the Overnights

The Third Night

Reggie was not scheduled to work nights again for another six months. A complicated pregnancy of a colleague changes all of that. Reggie detests the night shift. It is either real busy or incredibly boring. Time flies when it's busy, but either way sleep is disrupted. Although it is possible to catch a nap in the call room; it does not often happen. There may be a code called to resuscitate a patient who is non-responsive, or a nurse calling with a bull-shit question. Only on occasion do the stars line up and the passionate, petite Latina, Rocio, finds her delicate way into the spartan confines of the call room with him. It is during these interludes that he feels alive with a real mind and body connection and sense of oneness. This feeling eludes him otherwise. It is nice to recall something, taste something, smell something, feel something as his senses become alert and he feels alive and loved.

The night work and sleeping until the late afternoon messes up a normal routine. Everyday events such as shopping, mailing a letter, working out become more difficult. Meals become difficult to eat on time. Even finding time to go the bathroom is a challenge. Finding an unoccupied bathroom that is clean is a tougher challenge at times. Sometimes an empty patient's room is the only refuge.

He is in the drive through line at

the coffee shop, he hears a familiar voice through the speaker. It is the soft, melodic voice of Jill as she says, "Good evening, what can I get for you?"

"Jill?" Reggie asks the only red haired, blue eyed acquaintance he has.

"Reggie!" she exclaims as she smiles with her eyes and mouth. "Where have you been?"

"I got stuck working nights again," He replies begrudgingly.

"When are we going to a club?"She leans forward and smiles.

"Soon," he replies, "Soon, got any fresh coffee?"

"Absolutely!" she beams, "Especially for you, you're my favorite doctor! I got a riddle for you." She moves her head playfully, her ponytail moving about.

"What is it?" Reggie looks at her softly; curious about what is to follow.

"What is the difference between God and a doctor?" she grins playfully.

"I dunno?" he replies to play the set up

role as the straight guy. It's a bit of humor he has heard many times, but it's still relevant, accurate and funny.

"God doesn't think he's a doctor," she replies with a giggle.

Reggie serious facade breaks as he finds a smile pushing up his cheeks. He is still smiling after she hands him the fresh brewed coffee. "I need you to do a pelvic exam soon," she says with eyes directly meeting his.

"Just call the clinic, and make an appointment," He replies after feeling his lip warm from the cup lid, and enjoying a sip of his hot, bold coffee.

"Not that kind of pelvic exam!" She ostensibly playfully smiles and continues to look intensely at him. Subconsciously, she licks her lips, and thrusts her pelvis ever so slightly forward.

Nodding affirmatively and grinning he loosens the grip on the steering wheel. "She has the hots for me," he thinks. He returns the gaze, she gently caresses his hand as she hands him his coffee. "Thank you," he takes the cup slowly, maintaining eye contact with her. "I owe you one. I'll see you get your exam; real soon."

"My number is on the cup's sleeve. Give me a call; surely you can find the time to give me a call? My clinic can be open anytime."

Maintaining eye contact; she keeps it until he looks at her large text, neatly scribbled phone number.

From 7 pm to 7 am is the night shift; the sun is slowly approaching the horizon as he feels a warm breeze on his left cheek. He walks with his head down toward the entrance in deep thought. He has put in time at the clinic today, and may likely stay up all night. He dreads tomorrow as he will have to go to the clinic for a few hours before he can return home to sleep. He despises the transition from sleeping at nights to sleeping during the day.

Included in his rumpled, long white

coat is his walkman, some ear buds and a relaxation CD, just in case he gets the opportunity to sit or better yet lay in the call room.   The bustle of the hospital is subdued now as more visitors are leaving than arriving.

Journal Entry:

I remember hearing that much of the time individuals seek healthcare is due to psychological reasons more than medical reasons...there appears to be some truth to that...patients get an otherwise benign, even imaginary symptom, and all of the sudden they think they are dying from some exotic disease...or they have some psychological need to have someone take care of them so they make themselves sick...they have some idea that someone else is responsible for their health, because it's not up to them to take care of themselves...They actually think that they are automatically supposed to develop chronic diseases such as hypertension, diabetes, and any other condition as they increase in age. They do not believe they can take any control of their own lives and health. They think keeping appointments and taking their prescribed medicine is all they are supposed to do. I guess it's the 'best practice' for the disease management business that is the profession, but really, really bad for them. Intellectually, I know how this happens; as individuals give up their autonomy and trust outsiders to manage their lives...I also see how selfish, and self-centered they are as they use their medical coverage for bullshit visits or because it provides them an activity much akin to recreation; to go visit the ER. One patient, who literally lived across the street from the hospital; called an ambulance to transport her, when she could easily and safely walk!"

Moving quietly among the visitors entering through the smoothly opening automatic doors. His incognito cameo is interrupted by the blank, curious stares of patients awaiting to be seen in the emergency department. "Half of them probably don't even need to be here," "I guess theres not much good on the television." A smile on the outside is the only clue he is enjoying a private joke on the inside.

"Reggie, can you do the H and P on this new admit for Doctor Ayauasca? He's running late getting here from his clinic, and we're getting behind?"

The voice is from the ER charge nurse who is looking poised despite the chaos of the moment. She is an attractive, middle age woman, and apparently a cougar. She has a well earned reputation for indulging the temporary, carnal companionship of men under thirty years of age. Her personal preferences aside, she enjoys being a nurse and is very professional and old school. "There's some fresh coffee brewing in the lounge if you need it." She notices he appears tired as his shoulders roll forward as he stops suddenly and looks toward her; making sure he is hiding his frustration. "Sure, I'll be glad to help, but can you call unit three and let them know I am here, and helping the unit out? The charge nurse on the unit is a stickler for punctuality."

"Yes doctor, I know Anna, I'll call her now, she can be rigid at times. The patient is in room three, You'll find Miss Johnson with her son and daughter in law; she's been discharged recently."

Reggie sighs, and takes an informed glance at her chart. She is a seventy-two year old, caucasian female with a history smoking, type two diabetes, hypertension and congestive heart failure. She is taking fourteen different prescription medicines daily. Her chief complaint is shortness of breath. Vital signs show a pulse of eighty-two and a blood pressure that is 182/88. Her pulse oximeter reading was ninety-one percent and respirations were thirty-eight per minute. It appears she has gained eight pounds since the discharge eight days ago. He hears the family members chatting light heartedly with her. They don't appear to be too concerned about her predicament. She has been admitted and discharged less than a month prior. This is not good for business. Reggie enters the room and introduces himself while washing his hands. He notices the patient does appear to be pale. When he takes her hand, he notices it is cool and puffy. He sees her shins appear shiny and puffy as well; the soft, fluffy flesh dents and does not rebound from his touch.

"Mind if I take a listen to your chest?" It's a rhetorical question more than a request, but, as a courtesy he still likes to ask for permission before he exams a patient.

Her chest has the tell-tale sound similar to velcro separating. This indicates she is in congestive heart failure. This is all the information he needs to diagnose and admit her.

"Miss Johnson, miss Johnson..." he takes an audible slow, deep breath, before gently saying aloud while glancing at her list of medications. "This is a lot of medicine, you have to take,can you afford all of it?

"Yes doctor," looking up at him,

with dull eyes and nodding.

"Did you keep your follow up appointment with doctor Ayusasca?"

"Yes, doctor."

"Have you taken the medicines today?"

"Yes, doctor"

"Have you ran out or missed some doses?" He knows what her answer is before she replies.

"No, doctor"

"Well, ma'am you may need to be admitted to be at the very least diuresed, it appears you have some fluid on your lungs. I'll order a chest X-ray to verify the obvious. As far as being admitted; that's Doctor Ayauasca's decision to make."

Her son and daughter in law appear to be happy that she is being admitted. The truth is likely they are planning to be out of town and unable to find someone to stay with her.

It is not uncommon for family members or the patient to not take medications properly in order to develop symptoms and get admitted. It provides respite for the patient or family members who either want or need a break. Since she is a readmission with less than thirty days since discharge, the hospital will have to pay back the money received for her last admission. At that time she was treated and discharged after seven days. Needless to say, neither the hospital's business oriented administration or Doctor Ayauasca will be happy with this development.

He is absolutely sure she has not been compliant with her medicine regime, but that does not matter. After all the physician's responsibility to the patient is greater than the patient's responsibility to the physician. "I see you brought a bag of your belongings, I guess this admission isn't a surprise, huh?"

"No," she and her family reply in unison. Reggie thinks, "So, Miss Johnson can look forward to being taken care of for a few days, and her family gets a break, while the hospital pays back money due to readmission within thirty days of discharge."

"Let me check with Doctor Ayauasca to make sure that is what he wants, and to see if any other tests are needed."

Reggie walks to the physician's lounge, and grabs some snacks. He's not really hungry, but he is anxious, and anticipating some frustration from Doctor Ayauasca. He is procrastinating the phone call. He hopes he makes it here from his clinic. However, to be productive, and proactive; Reggie orders a CBC, a Chest Xray, and a psych consult to see if there is a mental health or cognitive issue to see if he can find another legitimate, billable diagnosis to make this admission new instead of a return admission. Intentionally, he takes a break to the bathroom, looking in the clean mirror and seeing the furrowing brow and tense jaw muscles in the reflection. He dreads calling him, "Shit, shit, shit" he says aloud thankful no one else is present.

As Reggie anticipates, the angry, frustrated, fuming, ventilating, at times incoherent, profane tirade of Doctor Ayauasca comes to pass. Reggie holds the phone away from his ear, because the volume is so loud, and penetrating. Doctor Ayauasca is a competent physician, and his frustration is in line with his indignation.

Understandably, he is frustrated and angry at the re-admission. However, he is pleased that Reggie is seeking another diagnosis and ordering tests to rule in another diagnosis. He tells Reggie to perform a digital rectal exam. This is to determine if there might be some rectal bleeding exacerbating the heart failure.

Reggie realizes that the rectal exam, while ostensibly appearing prudent, is likely punishment for noncompliance. It is obvious she is not taking her medicine correctly or more than likely is intentionally skipping doses. He finds a pair of nitrile gloves since he sees in the record the patient has latex sensitivity. With a deep breath and a sigh; he prepares for the pushback patients provide when there is an unexpected procedure.

"Miss Johnson, I have some good news and annoying news...the good news is you will be admitted..." He pauses to gauge the patient and families response; they nod, and are not appearing overly concerned, "The annoying news is I am going to have to check and see if there is some bleeding from your bowels...."

The family members look at each other and then at Miss Johnson who appears apathetic to the news. "Well, do what you need to do," She replies while rolling her eyes and then elevating her shoulders and releasing a sigh of her own. The family members wince, betraying their own discomfort with the procedure.

The tension in the room is palpable

and Reggie breaks the tension, "The good news, actually it's the best news is I have thin fingers."

Raising his hand reveals slender fingers. He hums dueling banjos. The reference solicits laughter from family members as he squeezes the clear lube onto his gloved, right index finger before gently inserting her tense anal sphincter which reluctantly yields.

The test is negative for hidden bleeding that makes another primary diagnosis less likely; she stopped taking medicine to get admitted. Miss Johnson appears relieved she is going to be admitted with the absence of rectal bleeding. She is relieved that she will be away from her family for a few days, they get on her nerves and she misses the life she had before her spouse died ten years prior. The loss of mental, financial, and physical autonomy is a painful ongoing event.

Reggie relays the news to Doctor Ayauasca whom surprisingly does not continue to ventilate his frustration. However, Reggie can hear the edge on his voice as he relays orders for him to enter. "Any other tests that you think might be useful Doctor Washington?" He asks in a sincere attempt to actually provide mentorship. "I trust you are thinking of the patient's interest."

"I would like to add pre-albumin, vitamin D3 and B-12 levels."

"Interesting, what are you thinking Doctor Washington? What are you looking for?"

"Nutritional status, perhaps there is a failure to thrive or diet creating health issues for her." He confidently says feeling the moment.

"Sounds like a good plan ," Doctor Ayauasca says, "Go ahead and order those as well. Good call, Doctor Washington."

Reggie cannot help but smile. He finally had a moment where is treated as a professional colleague, and not a robotic resident. These are far and few. He takes a deep breath and holds it. He wants to capture and hold this fleeting moment as long as possible. Memorizing the details so he can recognize it or recall it again. He reluctantly releases the celebrated breath as a sigh, respect feels good.

Journal Entry:

When I'm on, I'm on. I had two patient encounters that helps me feel like I belong in the profession, and gives me hope to ride out the shit storm that is post-graduate training. Both of them involved patients with psychiatric symptoms. The first; a 64 year old female with visual hallucinations reported to me by the nursing staff. She complained of seeing blood covered roses in her room, and under her bed. Not sure what to do, and treading cautiously with a new finding, I explore the situation with patient who is oriented to time, place, and person. She realizes that there are not likely blood covered roses in her room, but she sees them anyway. I had a lengthy conversation with her family. They report she had similar symptoms about ten years prior, and the doctors thought it was an adverse reaction to valium. The symptoms were alleviated when they discontinued it, and put her back on meprobamate. The hospital does not have the drug in their pharmacy, so I wrote an order to use home meds. Apparently, she experienced withdraw after about forty-eight hours off the drug, and the benzodiazepines do not replace the meprobamate; especially when you've been on it thirty-six years. Reading up on the drug, it was developed in the 50's for treating anxiety, and insomnia, and very popular, and addictive. Sad that she likely will remain on the drug for the rest of her days. Later that night and in the early morning, I received a call from the adult unit about an adult patient talking loudly to people whom aren't in the room. The nurse asks if I want to order an antipsychotic. I advise her, I better check her out before I do that. Being an orthopedic surgeon's patient we do not round on them, but apparently he is okay with someone else checking on her at two in the morning. Chart reveals she is post surgery less than twenty-four hours. I can hear her dialogue as I approach her room, and understand the nurse's concern. Her room is dark, lit only by the light penetrating from the hallway, as I enter, and introduce myself, I ask if there is anything she needs. She explains there are these ladies visiting, and they are keeping her up. I kneel close to her, and steeping into her world whisper, "And you don't want to appear rude, and ask them to leave." She nods affirmatively, and I continue, and whisper, "Don't worry, I'll ask them to leave for you." I then stand, look at the direction she had been looking, and announce, "Okay ladies, she needs her rest, so you are going to have to leave; now go." "Thank you doctor," the patient then rolls slightly on her side, and falls asleep. I guess something used in the surgery created the situation, but there were no more calls about her. The nurses, were very astonished, and asked what did I do to calm her down? My reply, "I put one toe in her world and kept my big foot planted in mine, I joined her delusion and then intervened by changing the circumstance." Not words I use, and truthfully, I'm not sure how I knew to do that.

<u>The Eighth Night</u>

The weekend without work's promise, of rest recreation, and rejuvenation, did not deliver. Being away from work, Saturday night and Sunday did not offer respite of his body and soul. He made attempts to catch up on sleep, rest, reading and socializing, but he is so tired both mentally and physically he couldn't effectively do any of them.

Saturday morning, he arrives home with adrenaline keeping him upright and conscious. Thanks to the idiotic traffic signals cadence, it is the longest, familiar four miles he could have drove to return home. Surroundings appear surreal and he has to work to prevent tunnel vision from taking over to navigate the twenty-five minutes of driving safely in heavy traffic laden with discourteous and careless drivers.

After dropping his keys three times, he finally unlocks his door. With a shove of the door, he enters the dark apartment, takes a deep breath, releases sigh and lunges toward the sofa. He gratefully allows the fabric to absorb him, and quickly becomes one with the furnishing. He looks at the clock on the wall with the little hand on eight and the big hand on three as his eyes close.

When the big and little hands of the clock are both on eleven, he sits upright and at that moment realizes he had been asleep. He has no dreams while asleep.

"Damn it," he thinks, "There is too much I have to do!" A fly on the wall sees the wide eyed Reggie with his hands made into fists.

Between the wrinkled, odor bearing

pile of laundry, and unpressed, clean clothes he feels overwhelmed. With the residential program's obligations, there is just not enough time for himself. He glances at the large pile of unopened envelopes that require his attention. He had plans to complete these tasks after arriving home, but fatigue got the best of him. He looks at them wearily and realizes he needs to get back to sleep, but the bathroom beckons him to take care of other priorities first. "It's so nice to take a crap away from the hospital, " he thinks as he takes a deep breath and enjoys the moments of solitude with the cool porcelain supporting him.

He nearly falls asleep on the toilet. The funk wafting from his arm pits reminds him that a shower is a priority. He has plans for the evening that do not include going to the hospital. He looks at the coffee sleeve with a number scribble on it. Not even enough time to hook up with an attractive lady; a smile breaks his face as he makes sure it does not get lost.

He has plans to eat real food! At a pharmaceutical rep sponsored event at a high end restaurant he could not afford otherwise. After the dog and pony show, and a medium rare filet mignon paired with a fine wine, he plans to meet friends.

The shower is welcome, and he enjoyed the luxury of not rushing, and actually savoring the cold shower. He lathers, rinses and repeats; feeling invigorated as he steps out and shaves the shadow off his face and neck.

He considers using the momentum to continue his day upright, however, the couch and sleep deprivation beckons him to return to the couch. Every other obligation needs to wait; he's beyond tired. He sets his alarm, because he wants to eat some real food this evening and not the gratuitous over-processed, sodium, sugar and MSG laden crap the hospital so graciously provides three times per day as part of their benefits. Tasty, but void of micronutrients.

The prospect of consuming real food invigorates him. However, the abdominal rumbling he hears, and feels now cannot wait. He finds four boiled eggs in a bowl in his barely filled refrigerator hidden among condiments. "This should hold me over until dinner," he thinks as he cracks the eggs, as he meticulously and delicately peels the shell before sprinkling some pink, himalayan salt upon their white flesh.

One at a time, he puts the whole eggs into his mouth and eats them like the hungry man is. Cold coffee is still coffee as he picks up a cup and uses it to assist the delivery of the protein to his tired, hungry body. Eyes heavy, the dose of caffeine has no impact on his ability to remain awake, as he finds himself on the couch and asleep within moments. Fatigue wins in helping him to establish his priorities for the afternoon. At five P.M. he awakens without the alarm clock. The rumbling in his stomach reminds him of the evening's plan. The glib optimism of the drug rep's dinner motivates him to get up, and dress himself with slacks, ironed shirt and polish leather the leather of his shoes. Within twenty minutes he is groomed, and whistling while heading out the door. Getting basic needs met is the top priority for Reggie.

He arrives at the restaurant's parking lot and notices another resident sitting in her car. He sees Doctor Kendra pouring what is clearly a clear liquid out of a half pint liquor bottle into a large cup, swirling it around, and lowering her head to the cup;quickly consuming it. She checks her look, and applies some fresh lipstick before getting slowly exiting her car.

"Oh man he thinks, she's getting a head start on the drinking." He's seen this before, when an individual who drinks before a gathering so they won't be seen conspicuously consuming a large quantity of alcohol while there.

He gets in step with her as he catches up to join her. "What's up Doc?" he startles her, and she pauses.

"Oh, hi Reggie!" she glibly replies as she quickly composes herself, "Are you looking forward to the dinner and dog and pony show presentation?"

"Absolutely, especially the informative, insightful presentation," he replies and she doesn't detect the sarcasm that accompanies the statement to her.

"Oh…yeah, I've heard good things about the drug." Still clueless, she pauses and adjusts her purse as she walks, careful to reposition and conceal the half pint bottle of liquid nirvana; just in case she needs a crutch.

"Really?" Reggie replies sensing an opening as he walks in step with her. "I've never heard of this particular drug…what are it's uses, uh, indications, side effects?" In reality, he knows it's a 'me too' product purported to be useful in treating the high systolic hypertension by removing excess sodium.

"Well, uh, uh it's supposed to prevent heart attacks and strokes?" She tentatively puts aside her contrived smile, and replies with a rising inflection in the pitch of her voice and replacing the smile.

"Thank you Doctor, now I can focus on enjoying the nice meal and drinks that they are so graciously providing!" As an afterthought he adds, "Be sure to take good notes."

"I will likely only have a drink with the meal," she responds with a somewhat defensive tone, "I'm not really a drinker...just on social occasions such as this, I don't have to have it."

"Right, right..." Reggie has to look away for a moment upon hearing her commentary, but composes himself and with a serious tone replies, "Good for you, good for you, a drinking problem is a bad habit to develop. It tends to sneak upon individuals slowly; as a matter of fact most don't notice it occurring, but others might."

"Yes," she replies indignantly, "It means an individual is weak, and lacks willpower! Some people just can't handle alcohol or any recreational drug. Smart people don't develop such problems."

Nodding in acknowledgement of her contrived statement, Reggie thinks with a great deal of surprise, "Damn…she really has a problem…unbelievable that she doesn't see it."

Reggie has noticed a double standard for the treatment of female students or resident physicians. The patriarchal foundations of the profession treats males with no tolerance for deviation from rules or norms; but are quick to 'rescue' the damsel in distress. The damsel quickly painting themselves with the victim brush of real or imagined oppressors.

Male attending physicians are afraid to lean on the females, because they know the woman's word will be taken over theirs if they suggest impropriety. In medical school they had the same luxury, and different standards. He often notices they are quick to play the gender card, a luxury males don't have. Even worse chivalrous men attempt to rescue them when they play the damsel in distress card. Although, they often describe themselves as strong and independent, they don't hesitate to play the gender card.

Ever the gentleman, Reggie walks ahead and opens and holds the door for her and some other patrons to enter. The sounds are background noise, and the aromas emanating from the inside, representing the plethora of food greeting his nostrils, are welcome. The cool air exiting the entrance is a welcome contrast to the outside's warmth. "I'm here," he thinks, "I have arrived." Squaring his shoulders, and raising his chin, he makes his entrance.

The well dressed brunette, dressing and acting as a cheerleader, and a real employee, of the powerful, influential pharmaceutical industry, is flawless in presenting the contrived talking points to the captive audience enjoying their choice of filet mignon, chicken, or the vegetarian alternative. It's business as usual.

Reggie is gently sipping his beer when he overhears a conversation as an internal medicine doctor in attendance is approached to be a spokesman for the drug. That is a perk of being a 'top prescriber' of their brand. The wine buzzed attending physician, Doctor Graft, can look forward to an all expense paid, island vacation and honorarium for his efforts. Prescription writing drives their business model, and the physicians are the employees they don't have to directly pay.

Watching the attending physicians in attendance drink more wine than they should and a transformation occurs. After consuming half a bottle of wine some of them are actually engaging and decent as the alcohol dissolves their hard exterior and masks their neuroses. He almost forgets their inept ability to teach and overbearing demeanors. He hopes they don't have any patient encounters tomorrow, and that they can make it home safely tonight.

Journal Entry:

I got some extra sleep today, it seems to have shaken off some of the fatigue for a while. I actually got a decent meal, and it was nice to see some of the attending physicians and colleagues loosen up with the help of copious portions of wine. I could not let my guard down let alone my hair down. I had a glass of wine, but don't require alcohol to numb in order to feel something; also I have to drive home! A colleague with an obvious alcohol problem certainly discretely, and efficiently put away more than her fair share. She didn't look intoxicated, but obviously was. I asked if she was okay to drive, and she got defensive. I want to say something, but it is not any of my business, unless in the unlikely event she asks me directly...Too bad they cannot be loose without the booze...I know 'experts' say addiction is a disease, and that they can't help themselves, but I don't think that's the only explanation; but it's the money making one!

The Eighteenth Night

Nurse Evans furrows her brow as she squirms in her chair. Ostensibly it's to get more comfortable, but the reality is she is uncomfortable disturbed by the physician's order she is reading. Sighing, she feels her pulse rate quicken, and despite the cool ambient temperature feels uncomfortably warm and notices her palms are sweaty, and her hands trembling. She rests her trembling, sweaty hands in her lap to maintain the illusion of poise.

She looks at the order again to make sure she is reading it correctly. "Has Doctor Washington rounded yet?" she asks to no one in particular.

"No, he hasn't rounded yet, but he's still the night resident so he'll be around." The unit secretary replies.

"Thanks," nurse Evans replies, "Let him know that I'd like to talk to him."

She unconsciously shakes her head as she reviews the order. "I can't believe he's doing this again," she thinks. Her mouth tightens as she catches herself clenching her jaw muscles, which bulge and her teeth to hurt.

"God grant me the serenity to accept the things I cannot change." Closing her eyes, she whispers this as a mantra under her breath. Her past in dealing with addicts and alcoholics helps her to read people. It's a skill that comes in handy for spotting bad intentions. Intuitive as well, she has a knack for picking up any bad vibes from individuals and situations. Her antennae are up on high alert.

She knows the unit. She knows the pathology and strengths of her staff. She knows the nurses that are likely to take the patient's narcotics. She knows the staff, and their biases towards working with certain patients or physicians.

Wounded individuals sometimes become nurses, because they are drawn to the potential for power, drama, and excitement. They often come from very dysfunctional situations, and sometimes enjoy recreating them in the day to day work environment.

The order at a glance, or to the uninformed seems innocent enough. It is an order to discontinue a calcium channel blocker. She has seen this before with others. It inevitably leads to an arrhythmia of the heart; first beating irregularly and ultimately cardiac arrest and cessation of life.

"Why is Doctor Morton doing this?" she thinks a furrowed brow is the only external clue that she is pondering the thought.

He is not the only physician who plays with medicines to the patient's detriment. She has noticed others prescribing previously used antibiotics obviously noticing they are not likely to be effective. She has seen opiates prescribed with doses that create respiratory arrest in individuals. She has seen living wills altered from full code to do not resuscitate without the patient's approval. Residents who don't want to deal with a code situation have been known to change them to accommodate their anxiety.

Ignorance might be bliss, but she is far from stupid. She can only grin awkwardly when she sees doctors elated that an elderly patient is admitted with pneumonia or a urinary tract infection. They are elated in the first few admissions as there is likely going to be payment for their efforts; however, after that they become their nemesis. The funds evaporate as the year progresses, physicians and hospitals despise treating patients for no compensation; it's a dysfunctional, but customarily accepted paradigm.

She loses sleep thinking about how nonchalantly that the physicians make those decisions that hasten a patient's demise. At one point in her career she rationalizes the patients had lived a full life, and turned a blind eye to the practice. Now she sees it as people playing the role of god.

This de facto euthanasia is not casually observed, but those with the discernment, and a knowledge of the pharmaceuticals pick up on the practice. Some physicians and staff take on the role of god more frequently than others; especially when they are no longer being paid for their services with the disparaged frequent flyers.

She likes the Reggie, he is not like the others. He lacks the ego, and know it all attitude of his peers and the attending physicians as well. He is respectful to the nursing staff, and even patient with the difficult patients.

She is torn about discussing some her current observations with him. Perhaps, he's noticed the same things, and she can ventilate to a compassionate ear. Or will he take her story to the hospital administration. She is so weary of carrying this negative knowledge; either is likely to be a relief; the weight of secrets is heavy.

She is relieved when she hears the brisk cadence of Reggie. She has easily acquired the skill of recognizing the sound of an individual's gait. She has been accused of having ESP as she announces someone's arrival before they approach the nursing station; she is simply aware.

She sits upright, inhales deeply, and takes a deep breath as she hears him approaching. "Good evening, Doctor Washington do you mind if I round with you this evening?"

"This is different," Reggie thinks. "I wonder what's up." He notices her discreetness, and sees her furrowed brow.

"Sure, who would you like to do first?" He says, assuming she may not have seeing everyone in mind.

"Misses Johnson," she whispers while stepping up to his side, and handing him her chart.

"Okay," he says as opens the chart. Upon close observation he notices she is on eighteen different medicines, is a frequent flyer, and eighty-two years old. "What are you thinking?" he asks wondering where the encounter is going. He opens the chart to new orders and glances at the poor penmanship to translate the plan of care. "What awful writing," he thinks, as he sees the new orders. "Let's go take a look."

Reggie knows her, and is familiar with the multiple admissions of Miss Johnson. A nursing home resident, she has exceeded the cap of reimbursements. She has been treated without the hospital or treating physician being reimbursed her previous admission and this one as well. She is typically laid back and easy going, but he is surprised by what he sees.

She does not look like herself. Her usual meticulous appearance is unkempt. Her pupils are dilated and she looks haggard. Her breathing is shallow and rapid and her frail, wrinkled, thin hands are clasped as if to protect her chest; she appears vulnerable and frightened.

"Miss Johnson, are you okay dear?" he asks to determine how aware she is.

"I don't feel well." She replies, "My chest is tight."

"Let me take a listen," Reggie says as he puts his stethoscope to her chest. Her choppy, irregular heartbeat, an arrhythmia is a new finding. He knows her shallow breathing which is rapid and high in the chest indicates a high degree of anxiety.

"Is your stomach causing you any problems? Have you had any indigestion or nausea?" he asks fishing for symptoms that may indicate an upcoming cardiac event.

"Are you hurting anywhere?" he asks as he attempts to figure out what is going on.

"No," she replies politely as she takes a slightly deeper breathe. "I would like to be able to rest," she adds.

Nodding affirmatively, Reggie says, "Let me see if I can help with that," as he and Nurse Evans move toward the door.

"What's going on?" he keeps his demeanor serious to hide his thoughts.

"Doctor Morton wrote an order to discontinue the calcium channel blocker earlier today, and she has missed two doses."

Reggie looks at the order and notices it is not supposed to start until the next day, "Well, the order is not supposed to start until tomorrow, lets catch her up, and I'll rescind the order; her heart beat is irregular, and that is something new he likely didn't anticipate. I'll order an EKG just to make sure all is okay."

"Okay," she says, "Thank you doctor."

"What in the hell does he think he's doing discontinuing this medicine?" he asks thinking aloud, "She has been on it for twenty years, and there are no adverse reactions with the current regimen. This doesn't make sense at all."

Nurse Evans bites her lower lip before saying, " I have no idea, but he does this frequently."

"Really?" his voice tone is matter of fact, but his inner repugnance is evident as he shakes his head, "I wonder why he's doing that? Either way, I'll write an order to continue the medicine, and everyone will rest better tonight… if she has difficulty resting, I'll add an order for melatonin five milligrams PRN, but getting back on the channel blocker back on board should help her settle down; and everyone will have a better evening."

"Yes Doctor Wilson, and thank you," she says as she gently touches the sleeve of his coat. She can finally take a deep breath and exhale a sigh of relief.

"She is due to be discharged as

soon as she is stable, why did Doctor Morton discontinue the medicine, did he make a mistake?" Reggie grimaces as he walks down the corridor to write the order.

"This is messed up," he cracks his knuckles, "Doctor Morton only has two admissions, and the other doesn't have any meds except statins, first line antihypertensives, and antibiotics...why is he discontinuing the calcium channel blocker? It doesn't make any sense."

"Well, she won't be dying on our watch tonight." he thinks as he takes a deep breath, furrows his brow, and notices tension between his shoulder blades. "What is that son of a bitch think he's doing!" Shaking his head and tensing his jaw in disgust. Feeling a wave of warmth envelop him; his breathing is becoming fast and audible.

"Doctor? Doctor! Are you alright?" Nurse Evan leans in, and touches his tense shoulder.

Reggie keeps his back to her and leans forward, ostensibly to adjust his shoes, but in reality in the moment, he nearly collapses. Composing himself he straightens up, looks at her and replies, "I'm just tired, it's been a long week."

"They have a tendency to drive first year residents into the ground." She places her hand on his arm, "Especially the good ones." She smiles and gently squeezes his arm while leading him to a chair.

Her touch awoke Reggie. It had been a while since he had felt a sincere, meaningful touch.

She sees a very tired young man with a good heart and good intentions. "Why don't you finish your rounds, and go to the call room and rest? I'll keep the staff from giving you bull shit calls. We'll save those for Roderick when he's on again."

Reggie chuckles at the reference, "I think I'm too jacked up to sleep." He attempts to move forward and she stops him with an upraised hand.

"Even if you lay down with your eyes closed, it will be better than hanging out at the nurse's station. Please, give yourself a few minutes, you've earned it."

It has been a while since Reggie heard warmth, and compassion directed toward him. "Thank you...I'll change the order, and deal with Doctor Morton later rather than calling him now."

Nurse Evans nods, "He doesn't like to receive calls after hours anyway. Now, go get some rest, I'll not let the drama seeking staff interrupt your rest! You've earned it." She walks alongside him making sure he is going to the call room. She senses he is on the edge of an abyss. He is visibly shaking, and her soft, warm hand finds it's way to his shoulder. His muscles are tense, his shoulders are elevated and his breathing is shallow, and rapid. He forces a deep breath, feeling his chest, and belly expand is a welcome sensation.

"Let me stay here for a few minutes and catch my own breath," She guides him to the bed, and he collapses on it. Pulling ups chair, and taking off his shoes, she begins rubbing his cool, moist feet.

"I know this may seem presumptuous, but I believe you need some touch to relax. By the way, I'm an instructor in therapeutic touch; it appears you need some humanity."

Reggie nods, and his eyes close. Her hands feel warm, and soft but strong. Within thirty-seconds he is drifting off too sleep. His body twitching as he continues to relax.

His relaxation is contagious as she leans over and drifting into her own rest, relaxes her back muscles.

He is so sleep deprived, he dreams shortly after she leans over his legs, In the dream he is walking along a stream. He hears the sounds of water flowing, birds singing and he goes to cross the steam, but the bridge only goes half way across the stream. This confuses him as the bridge had appeared whole just moments before. He turns around and is facing the same middle-aged man with a straw hat, denim overalls and scraggly beard framing a chubby face he has seen before. The face has bright, green eyes glaring through rectangular, wire frame glasses.

He is too tired to once again be startled awake by the cameo appearance of the curious, familiar visitor of his dreams. "Wh...What do you want? What's your name?" He asks with his foray into a lucid dream for the first time.

"I'm glad you're asking," He replies without speaking, in a telepathic exchange, as he pushes his glasses upon his nose with a pudgy index finger. "I am known as Maryan; spelled with a 'y' just so you know."

"Well, Maryan I've seen you before, many times, I'm glad to know your name...its curious you spell it with a 'y' instead of an 'i' so tell me how come I dream about you? What do you want from me?"

"I am not surprised you have forgotten," Maryan's look softens and he strokes his beard. "I am one of your guides; the top one of the hierarchy as a matter of fact."

"Guide? Hierarchy? Am I tripping? What do you mean by guides?"

"You have forgotten, but that is not unusual, because as a child you frequently interacted with us. You were delightful."

"I'm sorry to have forgotten, but what makes you show up in my dreams?" Reggie's inner dialogue is privy only to himself. The only clue of the inner work is the eyelids. Though they are closed his eyes are moving rapidly beneath them.

"I show up constantly, but it appears I am more of a distraction or a wake up all for you."

"Wake up call?" Reggie asks, "Like to literally awaken me from sleep? That's where I usually see you, just before I awaken, and other events as well."

"Yes, that is usually what occurs, so it appears now you are awakening," Maryan smiles,"However, you know there is more and there is less." His demeanor appears nonchalant.

"What am I missing here? I take it there is something I'm supposed to be doing, but I might not be doing it." Reggie watches as Maryan tilts his head, and smiles noncommittally.

"That is for you to recall, and decide. You are doing what you, and we, planned, but your freewill decides whether you continue with the plans or alter them."

"What do you mean?" Reggie asks as nurse Evans notices his brow furrow even though he is asleep.

Looking directly,and compassionately at Reggie Maryan communicates,"You can alter your path or continue with the current trajectory. Either choice is fine." Maryan adjusts his hat, tilting the brim up ever so slightly. "You need to wake up soon; and get back to your tasks."

"What should I do?" Reggie asks as his resting body stiffens slightly.

"That is up to you, and the course of decisions and choices. Remember, to remember, to remember" Maryan replies as he fades away in Reggie's dream as a Cheshire smile finds itself fading Reggie's dream. In reality only twenty minutes of clock time, and with a slow deep breath and even slower exhale; Reggie stirs around awakening nurse Evans whom had drifted off in her own rest break.

"Do you feel better Doctor Wilson?" "Yeah, actually I do, I feel like I started dreaming as soon as I closed my eyes. strange dream..."

"Lack of sleep does that; it can't be good for physical or mental health.

They can grind you residents under their heel without a second thought."

Reggie nods, and wipes his forehead for no particular reason with the back of his hand, "Yeah, I know, they want us to counsel and chastise patients about not taking care of themselves, but they don't take care of us."

"Doctor, after you finish rounding, stay close to my unit, I'll make sure you don't get inundated with bull shit requests for the new nurses."

"Thank you, I need to hit the books on board review anyway."

The dream and meeting the character who has been part of many dreams over the years is still fresh in his conscious thoughts. The dialogue exchange does not seem to be the result of a tired mind, but rather a meeting of the mind. The name, Maryan is not familiar to him, and it's strange that when he heard the name in the dream it was understood to be spelled in those words. "What did the dream mean? What did he mean? What did he mean by the plans going as planned and freewill?" Reggie literally stops walking as these thoughts quickly form in his awakening consciousness.

"Are you okay?" Nurse Evan's compassion rears it's attractive head again.

"Yeah, I just have to adjust my shoes. I'm good."

"You're our favorite doctor, and we got your back. We don't hesitate to defend you when the ignorant attending go fishing around for dirt. We protect you, but others are not so lucky. Roderick for instance has earned no respect from us."

"Really...why thank you," Reggie feels his skin flush as he is not used to hearing direct, supportive feedback."

"We have spoke to the attending about Doctor Kendra. We got tired of smelling alcohol on her breath as well as her obnoxious bedside manner."

"Really, what did they do?"

"Well, you know she is up Doctor Turner's ass. So she apparently doesn't believe us. She makes excuses for her, and accuses us for singling her out due to jealousy. When she was working the nights, we noticed that she was changing patient's living will preference from full code to do not resuscitate without the patient's consent, and we reported her activities to Doctor Turner and the medical education director."

The statement causes Reggie to stop in his tracks again, "Really, what happened?"

"Nothing, they backed up Doctor Kendra...The lack of common sense that so many doctors seem to have is not lost on nursing staff, the title of Doctor seems to go to their heads, and they can no longer be wrong."

Reggie nods, "I'm glad I'm not the only one who sees that happening; I don't feel like the lone ranger."

"There's a lot we see, and hear that goes on around here. It is so scary, If you know how many times I have seen the records in the chart changed, actually replace to cover medical mistakes...I don't recommend friends or family go here unless, it is something so routine...actually, I discourage them from coming here at all...not that others are that much different."

"This is a messed up situation," Reggie shakes his head as he looks down. "It doesn't seem to be about health at all."

"At least you're figuring that out early on, it took me nearly a decade to reach the same conclusion." She smiles and places her warm hand on his shoulder. "I believe Rocio is doing a fill in tonight, perhaps you'll encounter her during your rounds." You know, she's a friend of mine." She adds a wink to the smile she directs to Reggie. "Believe me, she is glad to hear you are on nights for a while."

Reggie feels warmth on his face, and an unintentional stirring in his briefs. He returns the smile, "Yeah, I hope to meet her if she's around, she's a nice person to hang with."

"I'm sure she'll welcome the opportunity! By the way, I've been keeping a list of strange practices by doctors, such as the incident you encountered tonight. It is more common; especially since reimbursement has dropped to the hospital from the third party payors."

"Its all about the money...just follow the money, and you can find the source of many problems..."

"Greed is the root of all evil." Nurse Evans seems relieved to be able to tell someone about her list of bad outcomes created by medicine changes. One or two times can be a mistake, or bad luck. Continuing the practice makes it a pattern.

Journal Entry:

I can't sleep tonight; even though I'm exhausted my mind is finally calm enough to write, but my heart is bathing in adrenaline. I overheard nurses talking today about a patient that had been transferring dying at another hospital; no surprise, for all intents and purposes he was brain dead when transferred. He was a tragic case where a simple repair of a prior umbilical hernioplasty took a wrong turn. It started with the surgeon opting to not intubate the patient; He chose this in spite of anesthesiologist's recommendation. Apparently the patient had contents in his stomach, and when the surgeon reduced the hernia, the contents of the stomach were vomited and aspirated by the unconscious patient; this is definitely not what the doctor ordered! Of course he is transferred to the ICU, and the chest x-rays reveal the obvious presence of pneumonia throughout the lungs. While in our hospital, he never regains consciousness, his lungs clear, and the incisions for his procedure look good, but he remains unconscious. I tell family members to assume he can hear them, and talk to him with goal directed conversation, and to play music or radio programs he enjoys. I can still hear Lionel Richie's hit, Sail On, playing in my head. I don't think the surgeon or the hospital was forthcoming about what happened. I reviewed the post surgical notes, and the entire narrative was different. On the first day, the surgeon's narrative was accurate about the events that occurred; the next day, a nurse brought to my attention the 'new' narrative. It was written in third person, and was completely different from the medical record's original narrative. The new version did not reflect any errors or misjudgment on the surgeon's part; just 'customary ways' and a bad event; and a convenient never before seen request from the patient to not be intubated! The day before patient was to be transferred, the surgeon, despite lack of a real need; as the central line in place was good for another ten days, inexplicably decides to replace the central line. It is not due to the patient's need, it is due to the physician's need. The surgeon, ostensibly to assist the transition, before transferring the patient can be reimbursed again for performing the same procedure. Remember, the mantra, procedures pay more! The hapless patient is eligible for another, and the surgeon was going to benefit from it. However, since he is being treated by the variety of physicians going in and out of the ICU there are too many cooks in the kitchen. The problem is none of them had bothered to look, or assume someone else had put the patient on anticoagulants. As a result, the patient, not being on any anti-coagulants at all, inevitably forms a clot. After removing the central line, and while

replacing it, an alert nurse notices the patient's oxygen levels drop to sixty percent. The surgeon assumes the tracheal tube has got displaced, and starts scrambling to get another. It is chaos as this tragedy unfolds. Eventually, the crash cart is there; all of the elements of a code are in place, but a code 'blue' was never called. I perform chest compressions, and feel the ribs cracking beneath my hands. There does not seem to be any life force left in him that I can feel. I see the patients' pupils are neither dilated or constricted which means there's brainstem damage. The surgeon barks at me to go faster, and I respond, 'I'm doing over a hundred compressions per minute'. Although the automatic electronic defibrillator advises no shock, the surgeon overrides it, and gets a shock anyway. The heart establishes a rhythm, but the patient is likely gone at this point. The hospital administration is glad to get him out of their (lack of) care. This case is a metaphor of the things that are wrong with the current healthcare system; anything that becomes profit first; like a fish rots from the head down. Another troubling 'practice' I'm noticing is what appears to be de-facto euthanasia. Patients, particularly, the elderly, and frequent flyers, especially when they have exhausted their annual medical care benefits have medications removed that create arrhythmias and ultimately death. I have seen antibiotics used that are ineffective due to antibiotic resistance for the patient. Often times the physician uses a different antibiotic drug from the same drug family used during an earlier admission. It looks as if something is being done, but in reality the antibiotics are ineffective, and the patient is likely to become septic, and experience septic shock and organ failure before they die. It is so dehumanizing to witness this practice of doctors playing god. They don't seem to be bothered by patients 'crumping'. Yeah, I get it everyone dies, but when someone sets up, and creates the death it's called murder. I occasionally hear them talk about how the patient has had a long, full life or their quality of life is going to suffer. All of these discussions have both merit, and appear to be poor rationalizations to justify manipulation of medicines to create their demise. Even hospice care, when they provide opiates to be used as needed for pain management at imminent end of life know what they are doing. It can be assisted suicide, or euthanasia. So many accepted practices are hardening the soul of medicine, and healing. It hurts my heart to witness these actions. It seems as if no one, other than a savvy nurse notices these practices. I wonder what the mindset of the physician making these life ending decisions is? What is also troubling is they make better decisions when they have medical coverage, and know there is going to be reimbursement. The whole system is disease management and not finding health, let alone promoting health or teaching patients to be healthy. That is much of the reason individuals find their ability to function decline to the point they are dependent on a profession designed to use them as livestock to make them money! Keeping them alive so they can make them money. Recently a hospice patient was referred to a surgeon for a procedure that would be costly in money, time, and follow up care, and the patient was in hospice! The ethical surgeon refused the referral, and suggested to the referring physician that such a procedure constitutes fraud! There has to be a better way of addressing health or regaining health! The current paradigm is primarily about making money for all the parties involved. I realize more and more it isn't about health, true prevention, empowering the patient or protecting the public. It isn't really about changing anything other than the amount of profits. I feel like a child seeing the naked Emperor marching down the street, and being the only one noticing he is naked. How do others not see what is going on? Do they even care? How can the unacceptable become acceptable?

The Nineteenth Night

Reggie enters the unit striding confidently. He does not notice any attending's automobiles in the parking lot. This generally means there will not be any pimping attending physicians or any of them interrupting his flow of rounding with their disrespect for his time.

Nurse Evans greets him and motions him to go to accompany her to the lounge. "Doctor Washington, I thought

I'd give you a heads up. Misses Jones was discharged today, and Doctor Morton does not notice the medicine order was not discontinued; he leaves a discharge order to continue hospital meds."

Reggie's brow furrows slightly, "I guess he didn't look too closely then."

"He didn't, but Doctor Turner reviewed the record, and was asking about the order change you made to continue the medicine."

Reggie feels his heart rate increase, his hands tighten into fists. "She did, huh." His nostrils flare.

"Yeah, I thought I would give you a heads up, she likes to 'drop in' and chastise residents. She can be a very, mean, and condescending, and a downright inappropriate bitch about the way she does it too. She'll do it in front of staff, patients or anyone else whom happens to be around." She shakes her head, "She is not very professional at all."

"That's all I need! For her to mess with me tonight." Reggie hears a ringing in his ears, and rubs the back of his neck in a visible display of the smoldering rage he is feeling within.

"My staff can run interference if you like..."

"Thanks, if you can do that; fine but if not, she really doesn't want to mess with me tonight. I'm approaching the limit of bullshit that I can tolerate!" Reggie's eyes narrow and his nostrils flare as he feels a hint of euphoria at the prospect of dealing with Doctor Turner." Feeling no fear, no fatigue, and he is locked in the frame by frame of the moment.

Nurse Evans sees a smile grace his face. "Either way, you have a heads up. We take care of those whom take care of us."

There is a lighter feeling in his steps and he is joyfully whistling as he rounded on the units. He hopes to meet the overbearing, arrogant, sell-out

attending with every step. He isn't
afraid anymore, and he is not hiding.
It is time for a reckoning. "Bring it
on," Smiling, he makes himself as
conspicuous as possible. He is tired. He
is tired of feeling tired being his 'new
normal'. He is weary of seeing human
beings being reduced to business
liabilities, and assets. His mind is
exhausted from his first hand experience
of the appalling lack of compassion in a
profession that has roots in healing.
His body is weary of the demands of
indentured servitude that immersion into
post-graduate education requires. The
sacrifice of mental and physical health
to fit your body and mind into a small
procrustean box. Selling your soul to be
a tool in a system that promotes disease
management instead of promoting health.

Reggie, always being the consummate
professional, continues his rounds. Once
again he is in a position to continue a
medicine that has been discontinued for
no apparent reason. He changes the

antibiotic on a patient in the ICU to give one of Doctor Morton's patient a fighting chance; clearly it is not an error that the antibiotic he replaces is not going to be effective again. His rectitude is still intact. This provides him an inner strength and fortitude.

He continues his parlous rounds and eventually while sitting in the empty cafeteria meets his reckoning. It's a physician who approaches him wearing an unctuous smile, and cold, baneful smile that morphs into a smirk.

"Doctor Washington, we need to have a talk."

"We do? Can it wait until I finish my rounds, I'm nearly wrapping things up."

"It needs to happen now!" She leans forward slightly at the waist in an aggressive stance.

"Turn around so I can kiss your ass doctor! Might as well get that part over with." Stepping toward her, he catches himself.

Doctor Turner's stance becomes rigid and upright, her arms fold high upon her torso. She cannot articulate it now, but she recognizes his fearless demeanor and gentle eyes that look right through her. "I don't like your tone right now, Doctor Washington..."

Reggie cuts her off, "Well I don't like you period! You obstinate, and obnoxious. You are no less than an overbearing, hypocritical, skank. You are creating a toxic work environment with your pure,unadulterated ignorance! So, I don't give a fuck what you do!"

"What! Now listen here..." She turns beet red, and her eyes are open wide as Reggie cuts her off.

"You are so ignorant, at so many levels that if your brains were atomic energy; you wouldn't have enough energy to blow your nose!" He has gone beyond the point of not caring. He experiences an out of body experience, as he sees himself talking to her. He continues his verbal cleansing.

"You are such a typical self-aggrandizing, selfish, narcissistic, mind-fucked, and full of shit doctor. I've had enough of you!"

Ever wanting to be in control Doctor Turner regains some of her composure, and with a dry mouth blurts, "As far as I'm concerned you've already screwed the pooch here!" Her face contorts into so much anger it causes Reggie to chuckle; seeing her lose control.

"Oh no, I'm so scared of the mean lady doctor" Cringing, Reggie feigns acting as a frightened child, all the while keeping intense eye contact.

"Judging by your actions and changing orders on the unit." She smirks, "You think you know more than a physical with forty years of experience practicing medicine..."

Reggie cuts her off, "First of all, the nasty son of a bitch has not likely changed the way he has practiced his so called medicine in thirty-nine years!

Secondly, he should not be playing god! He is murdering his patients whom can no longer profit him; or are you unable to see that with your head so far up his ass!"

Doctor Turner's breathing is high in her chest, and she has welts visible on her neck and exposed parts of her chest. "Well," she speaks through her clenched teeth." If you don't like it here then feel free to terminate your contract and leave. And by the way, so you know, the post-graduate community is small enough that everyone will hear about you; you smug little jerk!"

Reggie upon seeing her lose her composure, softly speaks, "Thanks for the invitation, you do what you need to do, and I will of the same. What goes around comes around, so you better watch your back! You never know when fate will greet you."

Journal Entry:

For the first time in nearly five years, I feel alive. I had an epiphany that played out, and now I am free of the bullshit that is 'modern medicine'. Fuck the overbearing, motivated by profit, self aggrandizing, hypocritical vocation masquerading as a noble profession. I am tearing away from it, and doing what I can to expose it for the bull shit it is. I remember going nose to nose with Doctor Turner, finishing my shift and terminating my contract with the hospital at 0800. Ten hours later, I 'come to' and find myself arriving home. I didn't drink or use any drugs that would explain the memory lapse, but there is a gap in my memory of about ten hours. I'm not sure what occurred, but my gas tank went from nearly full to nearly empty, but my car is clean, and my brakes don't squeak. I feel sore and stiff, all over, and my scrub's knees are stained with grass and dirt. I don't think I was involved in an accident, but either way something has happened, or I'm just realizing how sore, and exhausted I am. Also, I apparently got a huge basket of fruits and vegetables that I have no idea where they came from; and there's no receipt.

Regardless, I am glad to be out of that situation. It was becoming intolerable, and karma apparently has a sense of larger justice; the local television news has a teaser on an upcoming story of a missing doctor; their car apparently found abandoned in a bad part of town.

Epilogue

Reggie continues his meandering journey, driving around the city. Eventually, taking an exit towards a southeastern part of the county that is a bit more rustic.

A community composed mainly of German Baptists and Mennonites, and other folks, not associated with the religious faith, who like living simpler, rustic lives. It's a great area to find raw milk and fresh organic produce, and grass fed, free range beef chicken, and pork.

He notices the thumping from the rear of the car again. He takes a side road off the main highway. It makes a different sound underneath his tires as it is unpaved, and along rolling fences, and green countryside. He comes upon a small home and sees people attempting to manage a man who has apparently has lost consciousness.

"I'm a doctor! Can I help?" Reggie shouts through the window as he grabs his stethoscope. The older, thin, and elderly man has a week chin likely from decades of wearing dentures. Their profile is visible in his upper pocket.

"What's his name?" Reggie directs the inquiry to no one in particular as he deftly,swiftly,but calmly kneeling next to the man. The soft, short grass feels cool and moist on his knees; a relief from the heat.

"Levi" someone answers, "He fell asleep in the chair, and then fell down as he got up from it."

"Thank you," Reggie responds as he notices the man is not breathing, but has a weak, rapid pulse. A body that is struggling to get oxygen. He puts the fingers of both hands on the back edge of his jaw, and tilts Levi's head back.

There are two gasps. One of the gasps came from Levi, whose tongue extended forward in his mouth, no longer blocking his airway. The other gasp came from the onlookers, many who had been either crying or praying, relieved to see Levi raising up from what seemed to be certain death; and it likely would have been the end if Reggie hadn't stopped.

"His tongue likely rolled back while he was asleep, and blocked his windpipe. It happens sometimes." Reggie has binocular vision as the people around him seem to be far away. The many sounds around him become muffled, as he slumps onto the cool grass as exhaustion takes over; overriding the adrenaline, and cortisol he has been depleting.

Three hours later, he awakens, his shoes are off and next to the porch swing he has been lovingly placed upon. A woman in a long, floral print dress, and a pale blue bonnet brings him a tall glass of water fresh from their well. He sips it slowly at first unaccustomed to the non chlorinated taste, and smell. He then finishes it in huge gulps. Handing the glass to the woman and nodding when she offers to get more. Tired, and nearly dehydrated, he welcomes the cool water fresh from a well.

Sitting up, and noticing has car has been moved from where he left it. It looks cleaner than he recalls it being in a while. He looks across the yard, and sees a figure approaching the porch. It is a middle-aged man with a straw hat, faded, denim overalls and a scraggly beard framing a cherub face. The man is smiling at him with eyes peering through rectangular, wire frame glasses. As the man approaches Reggie, he can see the green eyes softly looking at him.

Making sure he is awake by pouring some cool water down the front of his chest. Reggie tentatively asks, "Maryan? Is that you?" thinking he recognizes the man as the individual from his many dreams.

Surprised, the man tilts his hat back, and peers at him, stroking his scraggly beard. "Reginald, how did you know my name is Marion?" Reggie can only muster a shrug of his shoulders; "Lucky guess?"

Marion nods, "I don't think we've met before, but I feel like I recognize you, even if I did get your name from your white doctor's coat. I do feel a bit bewildered, but regardless of those logistics, it is nice to meet you Reginald; your arrival is God's will."

Reggie chuckles and shakes his head. Adjusts his position to sitting upright, and on full alert. He notices his wallet is still in his pocket. "Yes, it is, but you can call me Reggie. And I don't know how I know your name, but apparently I got it from somewhere."

"I don't know either, but we are grateful you came by our way and saved Levi's life. You are an angel of our lord Jehovah, and it was his will to put you here today, and save one of our elders. The devil got his pound of flesh elsewhere."

Reggie nods, "I have no idea where I was going, it just seemed like the right road to take...But, I'm glad to be able to help. Is he okay?"

Marion nods, "Yeah, he's alive, and ornery as ever; he'll likely come around to see you in bit. We are grateful you kept the devil from taking him away from us! Pushing his glasses upon his nose. He points to Reggie's car he says, "By the way, I hope you don't mind us taking the time to clean your car, and taking care of the squeaking brakes, and the thumping noise that was coming from the back of your car." A hair rimmed smile, and a wink from a twinkling green eye punctuates the sentence.

Removing his hat, and sighing, he takes a brightly colored, but salt stained red bandana and wipes his forehead. "Doctor, I want you to know, you are welcome to come here anytime. You are different, and that is good. Perhaps you can find your way into our community. I got a good feeling about you."

www.ingramcontent.com/pod-product-compliance
Lightning Source LLC
Chambersburg PA
CBHW051916170526
45168CB00001B/409